I0765223

TAI CHI SWORD

Yang style
32 step Form

Juan Antonio de Blas

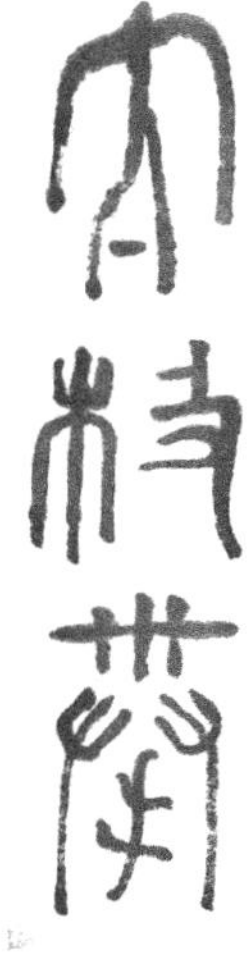

Neither the author nor the publisher are responsible for any improper use of the training techniques and methods described in the present publication.

First edition published 2021.

More info (in Spanish)
www.centrodantian.com

Aknowledgements

To Sifu Pedro Rico for sowing the seed
To Yu Bing Kan and Yu Wenching for the Art
To Marta Ester for the blue velvet
To Luis Gomes for the magic of theater

TABLE OF CONTENTS

...since water still flows, though we cut it with swords...

Li Po (李白, 701-762)
A farewell to secretary Shuyun
at the Xietiao villa in Xuanzhou

INTRODUCTION

* * *

The double-edged straight sword, called *gim*[1] in Cantonese and *jian* in Mandarin, is considered to be the queen of Chinese traditional weapons. Training with weapons in the context of traditional Martial Arts adds a critical factor of technical refinement; it consequently broadens the practitioner's knowledge of these disciplines.

Weapons training also adds an external element where to direct attention and intention. Besides that, adequate training in a great number of techniques included in the Forms with weapons constitutes a useful tool for personal defence.

The techniques of the straight sword are complex and subtle, and mastering them requires years of study and dedication. However, it is a subject that everyone interested in learning Tai Chi Chuan should know. This is because the sword, along with the long staff[2], is the original weapon associated with the development of this martial system since its origins, in all of its styles. The rest of the weapons that make up the Tai Chi heritage have been added over the years, coming from other Martial Arts or the adaptation of everyday objects for their use in combat. Of

---

1   Throughout this book, I use the Cantonese term *gim* to refer to the double-edged straight sword. This decision does not obey any concrete criterion other than personal preference. I use the noun in Cantonese, just like my Sifu taught me, as deference to my martial lineage.
2   The long staff, or *gwun*, is the grandfather of Chinese traditional weapons. They are usually made from white wax tree wood or rattan. It is a weapon of obligatory study in all Chinese Martial Arts. In the case of Tai Chi Chuan, it is frequent for the main long staff Forms to also be executed with a spear. In addition, it is also characteristic of traditional Tai Chi to use disproportionately long staffs for training.

course, this does not take away how interesting they are or their value; but, without a doubt, the historical and technical value of the straight sword transform its learning into an unavoidable task for any serious Tai Chi Chuan student.

Moreover, by contextualising the Gim sword fencing in the general setting of the repertoire of traditional weapons, we highlight the unique nature of its soul of steel, in whose heart lies the spirit of the dragon. This mythological creature represents, among other things, the ancestral wisdom, accessible only through Illumination. In the Martial Arts framework, the Forms and techniques of the dragon are, alternately, external and internal[3]. In other words, soft and at the same time powerful. Sudden but relaxed. Gracious and firm at the same time.

Also, beyond the martial scope, the Gim sword has a strong presence in Chinese culture. Through a symbolic language, embodied in numerous literary, dramaturgical and pictorial manifestations throughout history, the essence of the Gim sword is tied to the eternity of the Universe and the celestial Chi. It also bears a beautiful analogy with the subtle art of calligraphy, which is based on the delicacy and precision necessary to master both disciplines.

Lastly, it cannot be overlooked that, given that the geographical origin of Gim sword fencing is found in the mountain of Wudang, the Taoist philosophy impregnates every one of the techniques that forge the identity of the weapon. Thus, the hilt of the sword contains the essential human Chi, while the point of the blade projects the spirit of the martial artist towards the celestial dome. The straight sword represents the substance of the Tao[4], and, at the same time, treasures within it the greatest

---

3 Generally speaking, it is considered that Chinese Martial Arts are divided into two big categories according to their training methods and technical aspects that are given the most importance. Internal Martial Arts, or *Neijia*, are those based on the direction of the internal Energy and the harmony in the technical execution.
On the other hand, the external Martial Arts, or *Waijia*, base the progress of the martial artist on the physical event, granting a leading role to power and strength.
This differentiation can be relevant to better understand the methods of work that characterise, roughly, certain fighting systems. However, all Martial Arts balance both concepts and count on tools that harmonise this polarisation. Any martial artist that has reached an advanced level of training knows that the internal and external facets of the study are complementary and indissoluble. In any case, the fact that different styles have tended to evolve towards one or the other direction since their founding bears a relation to specific factors of cultural, religious and philosophical nature.
4 Tao literally means *way*, or *path*. Taoism was a philosophy before turning into a religion.

of martial refinements; in such a way that the harmony that hones its blade cuts the void with a stroke of evanescent silver.

This book describes, in a detailed manner, the 32-step Tai Chi sword Form of the Yang family. Through the pictures and the texts that accompany them, you will be able to learn the sequence and understand the execution of the techniques that make up the Form. Nonetheless, nothing substitutes the teachings of a good Master; for which reason, if possible, I advise you to search for a traditional School of an established reputation.

Apart from the description of the Form, the book includes some explanations and technical notes that aim to broaden the knowledge about the Gim sword and its use.

Through allegorical language, often mysterious, it advocates the individualism of the human being in communion with nature. Despite proposing ironclad moral principles, Taoism is a very open-minded and advanced system of thought

The Taoist postulates are underlain by a political and social reading of their time. Nonetheless, it contains ideas and concepts that, to this day, are still stimulating and innovative. Texts such as *Tao Te Ching* or *Zhuang Zhi*, become indispensable readings to understand the essence of this philosophical system, and are very easy to find in numerous editions.

HISTORY OF THE STRAIGHT SWORD

* * *

The Gim straight sword is indissolubly tied to the identity of Tai Chi Chuan, in all of its styles. Its origin, though, is much older. There are documentary records of Gim swords that date back three thousand years ago. However, these weapons were much cruder and more rudimentary than the contemporary swords, and their handling was also different from the fencing that has come to our days. These primitive versions of the Gim were weapons of war, wielded in very different circumstances from those in which, later, the theoretical foundations of the Gim's use started to be perfected. It is thought that the first Gim that bears resemblance to the parameters of the weapon we know today is the famous sword of King Goujian, found in Jingzhou, in Hubei province, in 1965. Even though this sword, forged in bronze, does not have the characteristic hilt nor the guard that make up later weapons, and it overall does not follow the guidelines for balance required by the exquisite technique of Wudang, it is a unique piece that constitutes a turning point with regard to previous findings. The sword gets its name from the sovereign that wielded it: Goujian, monarch of Yue, who occupied the throne between 496 and 465 BC. during the Spring and Autumn period (770-476 BC). This is the weapon of a king; for this reason, its rich ornamentation and the beauty of its forms come as no surprise. What did astonish the archaeologists responsible for the finding was that it did not present any traces of rust, as well as the fact that its blade remained sharp in spite of having been forged two thousand five hundred years ago. This discovery already denotes the identification of the straight sword with the elevated status of its carrier, and it reveals the effort undertaken by the craftsmen of antiquity to create superior quality weapons.

Other archaeological studies and pieces collected in numerous sites confirm that during the immediately following period, the period of the Warring States (475-221 BC), weapons of similar morphology but a much more modest making were used. With the passage of time, and parallelly to the assimilation of the straight sword as a symbol of erudition and aristocracy, and of the eminence they both often carry, the refinement in the manufacturing and use of more sophisticated alloys pushed the Gim to the pinnacle of traditional Chinese weapons.

On the other hand, and apart from the evolution of the sword manufacturing process, the elevation of the Gim fencing to the category of art is a process intertwined with the development of Martial Arts originating from the mountain of Wudang[1], among which Tai Chi Chuan is included. As already explained in previous paragraphs, the Taoist thought articulates, to a great extent, the narrative of the swords and their history. That makes perfect sense, since learning how to use a traditional weapon, in any context, always entailed embracing a particular ethical and moral code; or even, in many cases, a political ideology. This can explicitly be observed in the case of many Kung Fu systems, whose development was produced in close relationship with political and cultural changes throughout Chinese history. Also, in large part of the doctrine instilled to the Samurai through Bushido[2], in Japan. All of these matters might seem anecdotal and lacking interest nowadays; however, empathising with the way of thinking of those who created the discipline object of study, helps us to better understand its nature.

---

1 Wudang mountain is considered to be the cradle of the internal Martial Arts, or *Neijia*, evolved in the light of Taoist philosophy and cosmology. The most important ones of these disciplines are Bagua Zhang, Xinji Quan and Tai Chi Chuan.

2 The Bushido, or 'the way of the warrior', is a code of conduct that governed the life of the samurai in feudal Japan. The greatest treasure of a samurai was his honour, which allowed him to adequately serve his lord and the empire, the cusp of which was embodied in Shogun, the emperor, considered little less than a deity. In case of failing in his task, the samurai lost his honour, for himself as well as for his family. The way to restore the lost honour consisted in committing the ritual suicide known as Harakiri, or belly cutting. Due to the influence of cinema, manga and literature, a romanticised view of the samurai has proliferated, one that does not correspond to the historical reality in which the precepts of Bushido were formulated. Ultimately, this ethical and moral code had a specific practical sense in the context of the intricate Japanese society of the era, and served the purpose of controlling the samurai, who were the most powerful war tools of the feudal lords (*daimyos*), and of the Shogun himself, before the appearance of firearms.

According to an abundant number of records, the modern straight sword had an eminently ritual value, and its origins are linked to ancient ceremonies in the heart of the Taoist tradition. Nevertheless, and although it is true that the sword played a key role in this setting, it seems doubtful that this could be its actual origin in said context. Not only are there numerous documents that contradict this thesis, but also, we must bear in mind that swords, aside from the accessorial uses attributed to them in different circumstances, are weapons. And weapons have been created for one sole purpose: fighting. Further still, we must take into consideration the investigative effort invested in the study of increasingly lighter and more resistant alloys, with the purpose of creating impeccable blades. Even though the elaborate craftsmanship related to the embellishment of the weapon can indeed be justified by a ceremonial or tribal purpose, the evolution in the development of manufacturing techniques aimed at achieving more advanced weaponry responds to the desire to increase the probability of success in a situation of actual combat. In any case, these matters are not easy to clarify.

Following the trail of the documents and texts about which there is certainty, the analysis of the martial tradition of the straight sword leads, as already indicated, to the mountain of Wudang. Wudang straight sword fencing is a discipline in itself, independently of whether it has spread through the whole of China and has come to form part of almost all traditional Martial Arts. The origin of this school of fighting dates back five hundred years before the Ming dynasty (1368-1644), and the founding of the lineage is attributed to the mythical figure of the erudite Zhang Sang-Feng[3]. According to this version of events, the most widespread and accepted one, Master Zhang tutored nine disciples, who in turn founded nine martial branches. Three of them dedicated their work to the development of internal empty hand systems, three to the handling of knives, and three others devoted their efforts to straight sword fencing. One of these three schools was the famous Dan sect (Dan Pai), root of contemporary fencing. The Master who started the lineage of this particular

---

3   Zhang Sang-Feng is a very relevant figure in Chinese culture. The specific facts of the biography of this acupuncturist, erudite and warrior are diluted in legend. He was born during the last decades of the 13th century, probably before the fall of the Song dynasty (960-1279). The creation of the sequence of the thirteen movements of the original Tai Chi Chuan, the refined art of Dim Mak, or 'death-point striking', and the founding of the lineage of the double-edged straight sword fencing, are all attributed to him.

branch was Zhang Song-Xi. Over the years, the teachings of this school enjoyed great expansion, in great part thanks to the wandering monks who travelled throughout the territory, teaching the precepts of the Tao and its inherent rites. However, the cloak of the guardian of the style always fell on the shoulders of a Taoist monk. This tradition was broken in the eighteenth generation when Grandmaster Zhang Ye-He considered that the martial ability of his most notable disciple, Song Wei-Yi, was more important than preserving the custom. Thus, Grandmaster Song inherited the secrets of the Dan Pai, and Wudang fencing achieved renewed notoriety across the whole of China.

It is necessary to highlight the fact that the peak of Wudang fencing during the early stages of the 20th century is contingent on the will to exalt all Martial Arts to present them as an identity symbol of the Chinese nation. In the case of the straight sword, it was also deemed necessary to dissociate the weapon and its techniques from artistic and cultural manifestations deeply rooted in the collective memory of the Chinese people. At the same time, sharpening the blades of those swords that had a mere testimonial value, linked so much to the social position as well as the philosophical, ethical and moral patrimony of a whole nation, became an inescapable task. Understanding this context helps satisfactorily explain the determination with which the Masters of Wudang fencing gave themselves to the task of reclaiming the sublimity of their Art.

Everything presented in this part of the book contributes to clarifying many of the reasons why the straight sword plays such a key role in the Tai Chi Chuan panoply. In summary, it is a process that has to do, on the one hand, with the development of the martial discipline of the straight sword in the heart of the Taoist order of Wudang, and, on the other hand, with the spread of the techniques by the Dan Pai. In concrete, general Li Jinglin, known as China's first sword, a disciple of Song Wei-Yi and Master of the nineteenth generation of the lineage of Wudang, was a determining figure that synthesised and disseminated the technical content of the work with the straight sword throughout China. In the case of Yang style Tai Chi Chuan, Wudang fencing is linked to the techniques of the system through the relationship between Li Jinglin and Grandmaster Yang Chengfu[4]. Despite the fact that general Li

---

4　Yang Chengfu (1883-1936) was the grandson of the founder of Yang Tai Chi Chuan, Yang Luchan the Invincible (1799-1872). He was the one responsible for the systematisation

became interested in Tai Chi Chuan thanks to Yang Chengfu's uncle, Yang Jianhou (1839-1917), it was his close friendship with Yang Chengfu that permitted him to bring the two disciplines together.

According to the explanations of Chen Weiming[5] in his famous treatise, Yang Chengfu never taught a specific Form of the straight sword, but, rather, the classic Form of fifty-five steps was put together based on free practice and the refinement of isolated techniques and sequences. This fact may seem strange from the point of view of many martial artists versed in other disciplines; however, free practice, also known as sword dance, *Wu Jian*, is considered a method of advanced training of Wudang fencing; being, on top of that, from a philosophical point of view, an idea very characteristic of the Taoist thought.

In our lineage, this joint tradition was distilled and passed down by Grandmaster Hu Yuen Chou[6]. It is so because Grandmaster Hu, one of the most reputable experts in the field of Chinese Martial Arts, had the opportunity to learn behind closed doors from both Chen Weiming and Yang Chengfu, as well as from general Li Jinglin himself. Without a doubt, the technique of the Wudang straight sword is one of the many treasures that Hu Yuen Chou's wisdom has contributed to our lineage; not only in the case of the Tai Chi sword, but also in that of Kung Fu Choy Li Fut. Nowadays, these teachings are still alive through the labour of Grandmaster Doc Fai Wong, a direct disciple of Hu Yuen Chou.

---

of the style through the creation of most of the original Forms and his painstaking and continuous educational work, until the end of his days.

5   Cheng Weiming (1881-1958) was one of Yang Chengfu's most outstanding disciples. A man of profound knowledge, he had the will to put together the teachings of his Master in writing, and from his quilt spring the first books that expound the key principles of Yang Tai Chi Chuan in a didactic way.

6   Grandmaster Hu Yuen Chou (1906-1997), also known as Woo Van Cheuk, has gone down in the history of Chinese Martial Arts as one of its greatest exponents. He was a wise man who dedicated his long life to spreading Martial Arts and bringing together the different traditions in a comprehensive and consolidated compendium of knowledge. Grandmaster Hu represents a nexus with the original Sifus, and, thanks to his ecumenical mentality, he became the catalyst for the subsequent knowledge. To a large degree, all Chinese Martial Arts practitioners we are indebted to his generosity and vision of the future.

PARTS OF THE GIM SWORD

*** * ***

In order to better understand the techniques that define the handling of a given weapon, it is essential to get to know its structure and characteristics. In the following illustration, the reader can see the different parts into which the straight sword is divided.

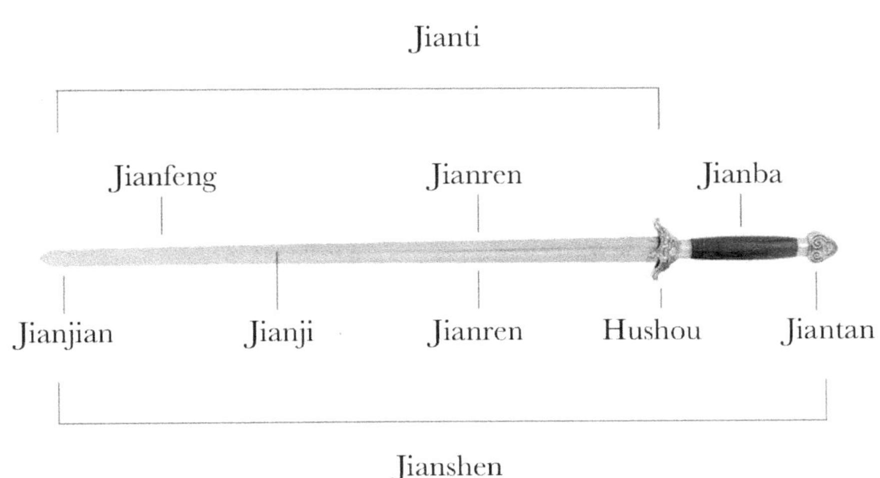

SOME TECHNICAL NOTIONS

* * *

Before tackling the study of the sword Form that gives title to this book, it is opportune that you become familiar with some of the key concepts about its handling. As already shown in the introduction, the technique of the Gim sword is extremely complex and, from a functional point of view, its learning requires specific instruction from a qualified Master. Nevertheless, and beyond a concrete analysis of the Form and the techniques that comprise it, the knowledge of the basic theoretical principles inherent to straight sword fencing contributes to interiorising the knowledge about the weapon and diving further into the comprehension of its practical application.

Besides that, regarding the general fundamentals that make up the technique of Tai Chi Chuan, this work is written from the premise that you are familiar with the theoretical and practical rudiments of Tai Chi; in particular, with its basic stances and steps. In all Martial Arts, stances constitute the root from which, with time and effort, martial excellence blossoms. In the case that you do not have any previous knowledge about the basic technical work in Tai Chi Chuan, the pictures that illustrate the Form will constitute sufficient reference. However, I recommend the manuals *The essence and applications of Taijiquan* (Yang, Chengfu. 2005. Berkeley, California. Blue Snake Books) and *Mastering Yang style Taijiquan* (Fu, Zhongwen. 2006. Berkeley, California. Blue Snake Books) as a first contact with the basic principles of Yang Tai Chi Chuan. Despite the existence of innumerable modern publications that discuss and elaborate on this matter, drawing upon the original sources always gives a deeper and more genuine view of the Martial Art. In any case, and beyond the basic concepts, in a later section of the book I will give some specific guidelines that all practitioners need to know.

GRIP OF THE SWORD

In martial practice, it is crucial to know and keep in mind the idea of the focus. This concept refers to the intention that the martial artist imprints on each technique. From this standpoint, the practice acquires substance thanks to the internal Energy, the Chi, of the performer. This principle is also an element of great importance in the cultivation of the *jin*[1], in the absence of which the techniques turn into mere lifeless movements. Consequently, the sword should be considered an extension of the will itself, and not a crude inanimate instrument. From all this, it can be deduced that there is a great difference between grabbing a weapon and wielding it.

It is common for beginners, and also those who, for whatever reasons, have learnt to handle the sword without taking into consideration the spirit of the Martial Art, to hold it by closing their hand over the hilt as if it were a simple stick or a similar object. This constitutes a grave mistake that renders the correct execution of the majority of the techniques impossible. The sword must be held with the middle finger, the ring finger and the thumb, leaving the index finger relaxed near the guard. In this way, the wrist can perform the precise and controlled movements that fencing with the Gim requires. This grip has some nuances depending on a number of factors, and there are obviously some exceptions as well, in specific techniques where the part of the blade closest to the guard intervenes, as in the case of the *Block and Sweep* techniques (page 61).

---

1   The *jin* is an inherent element in all Chinese Martial Arts. It is a concept that refers to the internal strength of the martial artist that can be transformed into power. The cultivation of the *jin*, through diverse training methods, has as its purpose the conscious development of the internal Energy, or Chi, for its application in combat.

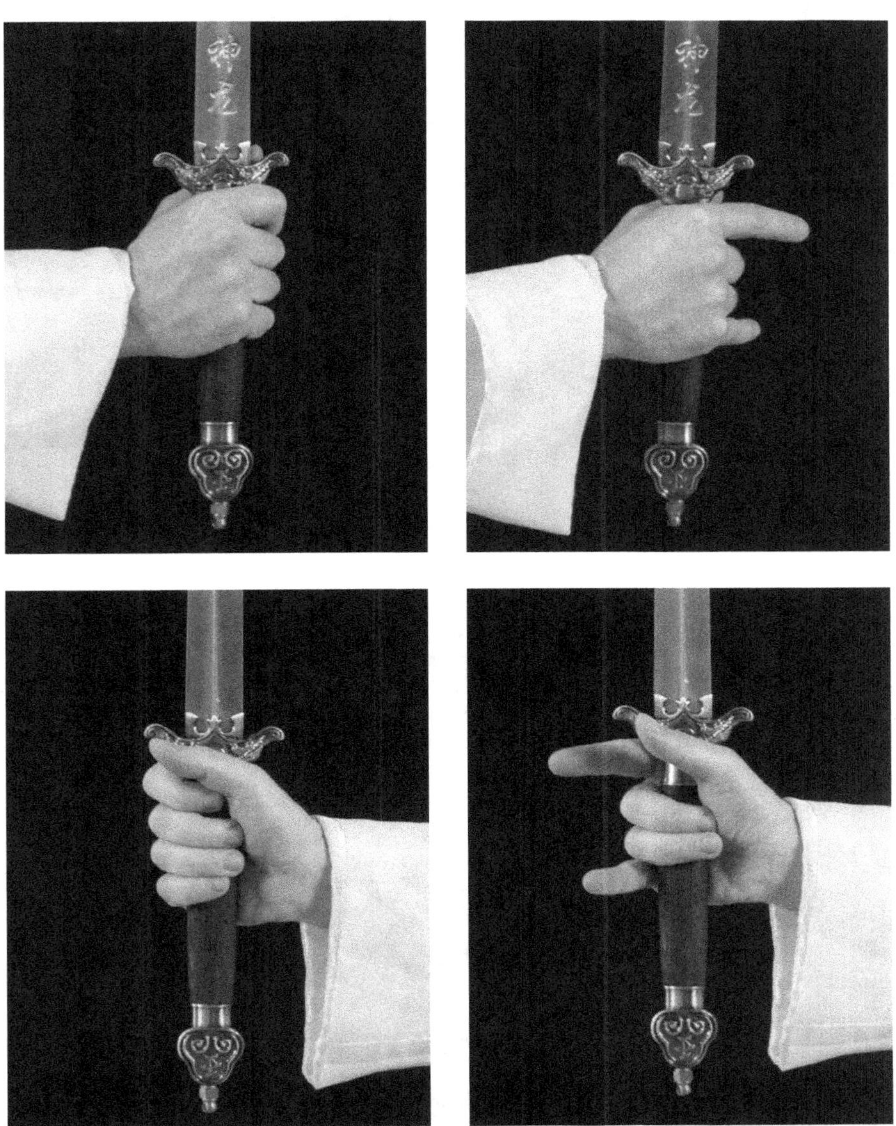

Correct grip

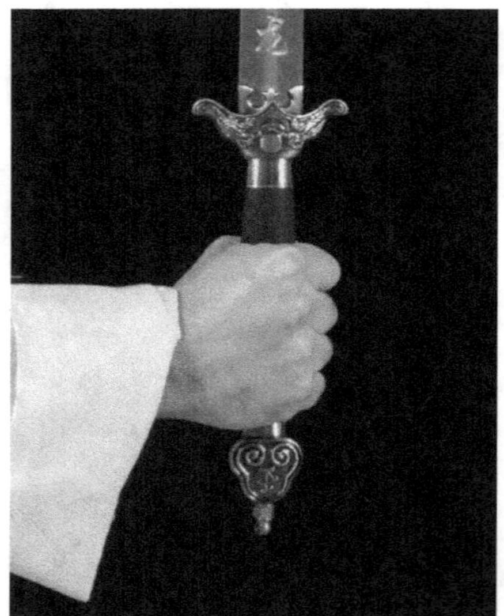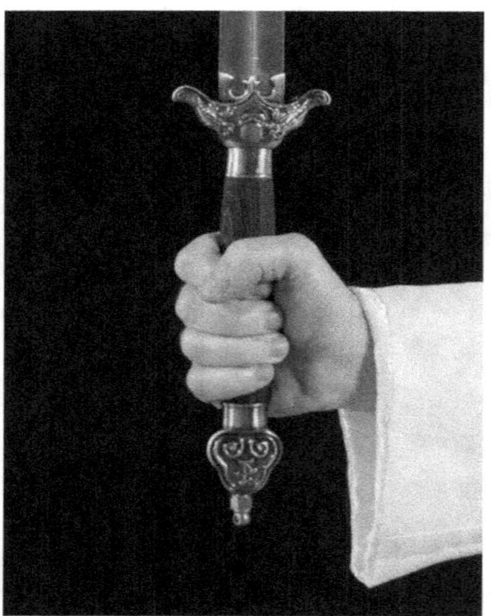

Incorrect grip

For example, the following picture shows the correct grip to perform the technique *The great star of the Literary God* (page 54). In this case, the general norm varies in order to add precision to the thrust. There exist more circumstantial modifications according to the demands of other techniques; however, the guidelines presented in the previous paragraph are the option that should be considered as a reference.

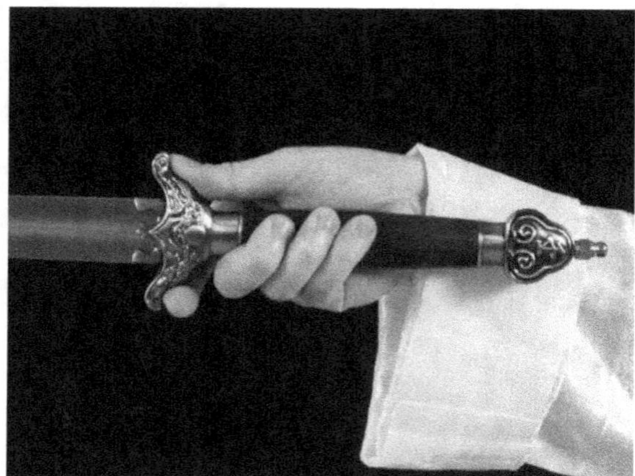

In addition, the design of the straight sword allows the martial artist to vary the angle of impact of the cut by rotating his/her wrist. This can happen at the beginning of a technique, or at some point during its execution. To facilitate the orientation during the study of the different techniques, the reader should familiarise with two of the traditional terms that are used recurringly to refer to the angle that the sword blade forms in terms of the ground. Throughout the description of the Form, the word *zhimian* will be used to indicate that the sword blade is vertical to the ground, and *pingmian* in the case that this is found in a horizontal position.

SECRET SWORD

One of the technical elements that characterise straight sword fencing, in all martial systems, is the so-called *secret sword* (shou nei jian jue), or *sword fingers*. The hand that is not holding the sword is always found forming a circle with the ring finger, the pinkie finger and the thumb. The correct way to form this figure consists in resting the thumb against the distal phalanx of the ring finger and the pinkie finger. The index finger and middle finger must stay together and extended.

This secret sword of an invisible hilt plays a central role in the execution of the techniques, since it contributes decisively in conserving balance, and it keeps the free hand away from the trajectory of the sharpened blade of the Gim. With practice, the student will discover the numerous nuances of the secret sword, whose position and angle determine the effectiveness of the diverse cuts, deflection techniques and thrusts.

In the case of the 32-Step Tai Chi Form, the secret sword is placed at different points, applying the criteria of the passive defence[2] positions used in the empty hand technique. Nevertheless, in many techniques, the potential functionality of the left hand is sacrificed in favour of speed and

---

2   In the correct execution of any martial technique, the whole body always intervenes. Otherwise, the harmony of the technique is broken, and its effectiveness is drastically reduced. On many occasions, the hand, the fist, or the forearm that do not strike are strategically positioned to provide an additional element of protection for the martial artist. Thus, it is frequent to see in several techniques the hand that fulfils this purpose close to the elbow or above the head.

balance. In the description of the Form, general indications will be given to complement the visual reference provided by the pictures. To understand the subtleties inherent to the precise use of the different secret sword positions, the practitioner needs to have received specific martial instruction.

JOINT RELAXATION AND VALUE OF THE STANCE

Working with weapons greatly contributes to refining the martial technique and improving all aspects of practice. In the case of the Gim sword, not only the solidity of the stance, but also the dynamic harmony in the execution of the movements acquire great importance. As it is an intricate and subtle discipline, it requires that the kinetic chain that starts from the stance be exempt from tension and imbalance. The stance should always be solid but light, and the muscle groups involved in each of the movements must remain relaxed, flowing towards the tip of the sword. It is vital to avoid postural tensions and breaking the natural geometry of the body.

The bow stance, which is the basis of the dynamic work in Tai Chi, is used systematically in this Form. Some static techniques are executed on the middle step that is frequently employed between two consecutive bow stances. Also, in the case of certain thrusts, the practitioner stands with his/her feet joined together, or balancing on one leg. Regarding weight shifts, some parts of the text that describe the Form indicate the necessity to put the weight of the body on one leg before initiating a displacement or carrying out a technique; it is a simplified way of saying that the weight of the body should be distributed between both legs in a proportional relationship of approximately 20%-80%, or 25%-75%. It is a resource that employed regularly to avoid, through the synthesis, that the text should become unnecessarily cumbersome and repetitive.

Moreover, throughout the description of the Form, on many occasions, I refer to the turn of the waist that accompanies the majority of the techniques. In this sense, the term waist is usually offered as a translation of *yao* in various languages, including English. Despite the fact that habit has eventually turned these two words into acceptable synonyms, the word *yao* does not only allude to the waist, but it also includes the lumbar spine and the lower abdomen, where the lower Dan Tian[3] is lodged. In Tai Chi Chuan, the rotation of the waist during the execution of most of the techniques is of vital importance; since, apart from transmitting power from the position to the contact point, this rotation also produces the internal massaging of the organs as a collateral benefit.

It is also necessary to establish the difference between two stances that, even though they have a similar appearance, fulfil different functions. It is a matter that frequently gives rise to misunderstandings that lead to incorrect technical execution. In various passages of the Form, the reader can observe how the displacement is produced by bringing the back leg forward, passing it in front of the other leg in a crossed step, in such a way that, at the end of the movement, the feet are at a ninety-degree angle and the knee of the back leg rests on the gastrocnemius of the front leg, which supports almost the totality of the body weight. This stance is very common when working with weapons in Tai Chi, and is also present in other Chinese Martial Arts. Its generic name is *quai ma*. Additionally, when the practitioner simply pivots on the heel of their front foot without a displacement being produced, leaning the knee against the back leg upon the calf just the same, it is called *nau ma*. The purpose of this second stance is not to move forward, but to obtain a wider turn of the waist avoiding loss of balance. This nomenclature is common to a large number of Chinese martial systems, and its use in the book contributes to establishing a clear distinction between the two stances. Also, it is a small indulgence that introduces the idea that, broadly speaking, the majority of Martial Arts share the same root.

INTENSITY AND SPEED CHANGES

During the early stages of training, it is advisable to execute the Forms slowly and smoothly, maintaining a natural and relaxed rhythm of breathing. From this point of view, the Form evolves as a sole movement,

---

3   Literally *elixir field*, Dan Tian is an essential centre to cultivate the internal Energy (*qi*, or *chi*), in the human body according to the Chi Kung tradition. There are principally three Dan Tian: the lower Dan Tian, the middle Dan Tian and the upper Dan Tian. These three energy centres are of critical importance in the processes that take place in the eight extraordinary vessels of Chi, the twelve main channels and their corresponding associated channels.

regardless of whether there are pauses throughout the sequence, either arbitrary ones or according to the guidelines. In the light of this approach, the beginner gains control over the most important principles of the technique, comes into contact with his/her own Chi, and can experience the essence of Tai Chi Chuan in the context of a pleasant and healthy practice.

Thus, it is correct to perform the sword Forms adopting this perspective. Nonetheless, if the student wishes to go deeper into the martial aspect of the sequence, he/she must learn to apply the exact intensity that each technique requires, and also to modify the speed in the passages where certain movements take place, such as, for example, feints and thrusts. In my opinion, this specialised work demands, unfailingly, the supervision of a Master. Otherwise, the technique will be dramatically devalued. For this reason, I advise you to practise the Gim sword Forms following the general guidelines that I have described in the first part of this commentary, unless you have the opportunity to take classes at a qualified Martial Arts School.

In any case, working with the straight sword, always bearing in mind the capabilities and needs of each practitioner, provides an additional ingredient that enriches the learning of the Art of Tai Chi Chuan. Even if we approach the technical analysis through relatively superficial levels of reading, studying the Gim sword always gives back a considerable benefit.

THE THIRTEEN TECHNIQUES OF WUDANG

Wudang fencing is based on thirteen principal techniques that serve as a starting point for the development of the entire technical repertoire. Naturally, there are many more techniques and variations of these techniques. However, general Li Jingling chose thirteen in particular because he considered they were the most representative ones of the style. He also chose the number thirteen to establish a parallelism with the thirteen primal techniques of Tai Chi Chuan. In the case of both martial disciplines, the fact that the essential techniques are thirteen is explained by the influence of the Taoist thought on their development. Thus, there are eight techniques linked to the eight trigrams described in the *I Ching*, or *Book of changes*, and five related to the Five Elements, *Wu Xing*, which determine the nature of matter in the Tao cosmology. The thirteen fundamental techniques of Wudang fencing, also present in the 32-Step Form, are the following:

Chou: draw	Dai: carry
Ti: lift	Ge: parry
Ji: strike	Ci: stab
Dian: point	Beng: bend
Jiao: stir	Ya: press
Pi: chop	Jie: intercept
Xi: slide	

THE SPIRIT OF THE DRAGON

This concept is mentioned in the introduction of the book as a poetic addition to the text, relating the symbolism of the dragon figure to the broader context of Chinese culture, but also to that of Martial Arts in particular. Nevertheless, beyond the rhetorical scope, this is an issue that deserves further elaboration, which corresponds to this part of the book since it is dedicated to specific technical aspects. The repeated allusion to the dragon as the soul of the straight sword is a metaphor that has a specific meaning applicable to the technique. The Gim sword and the martial artist must be one. In other words, through the quest for the perfect execution of each movement, the consummate swordsman reaches martial illumination, elevating his/her spirit, his/her *Shen*[4], and achieving, as a consequence, a perfect symbiosis with the weapon. It is in this state that the martial artist exhibits the long-awaited golden gaze and can perform the authentic Sword Dance, Wu Jian.

---

4   It is one of the Three Treasures *(San Bao)*, fundamental in the theory of traditional Chi Kung. The *Shen* is equivalent to the spirit and is divided into *Xin*, the emotional mind, and *Yi*, the rational mind. If the reader want to learn more about this and other concepts related to the Chi Kung, I recommend the works of doctor Yang Jwing-Ming.

HOW TO CHOOSE A SWORD

Firstly, it should be stressed that anyone practising Martial Arts has the responsibility to become informed about the laws that regulate the possession and use of weapons.

In the case of acquiring a training Gim sword, it is not necessary to invest huge sums of money in weapons manufactured with high-quality alloys or expensive ornaments. In fact, it is possible to get acceptable quality Gim swords made from aluminium or steel, at an affordable price. It is fundamental, though, that the weapon chosen should be well-calibrated. To determine this issue, simply lay the sword flat upon the index and middle fingers at one-third of its length from the pommel. If the sword remains straight, it is a suitable weapon.

There is also the possibility to use wooden replicas to practise. It should be noted that this is not necessarily a cheaper alternative. On top of that, it is much more difficult to correctly calibrate a wooden weapon, unless you make it yourself or commission it to a craftsman. In any case, wooden swords are used frequently in the majority of Martial Arts Schools.

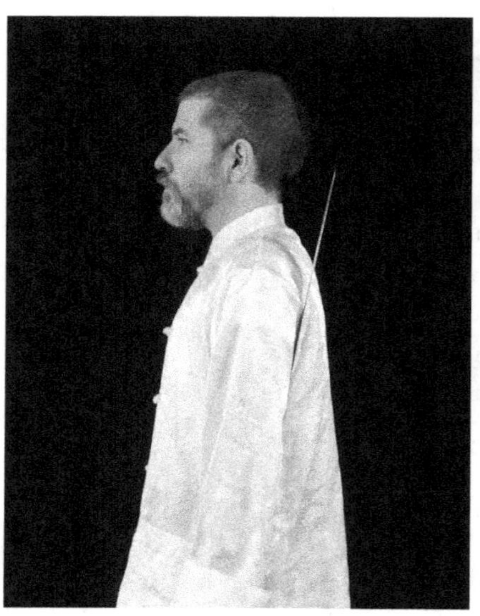
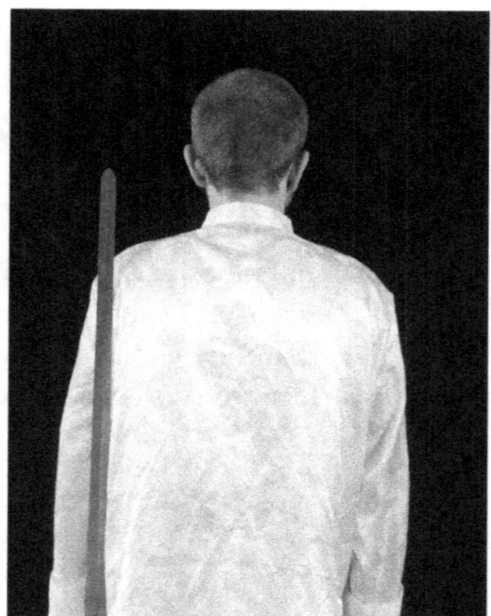

When it comes to size, it is usually determined by holding the sword with the hilt down and keeping the arm extended, so that the blade rests flat behind the forearm. Once we have the weapon in this position, called *fanwo,* the point of the blade should not exceed the upper part of the auricle.

Before closing this section, I find it useful to tackle a controversial issue that often causes confusion, especially among beginners: Are Gim swords flexible? It is true that the old swords, the evolution of which gave us as a result the Gim we know today, were rigid weapons. However, modern straight swords are semi-flexible. This does not mean that they can be folded like paper, but that their design allows the fine steel blade to vibrate when it hits a resistant object, thus avoiding that it breaks. In other words, a rigid blade as thin and light as those of the majority of the Gim swords would inevitably snap in almost any situation of actual combat. The controversy arises from the ambiguity between functional weapons and those designed for artistic and athletic display. The weapons destined for exhibitions are usually made of aluminium alloys, since the objective is for them to be manageable and light to attain more speed when executing the Forms. The confusion begins when one examines a display weapon using the scrutinous criteria that would be used for a real sword, an analytical exercise that lacks sense. This is something that does not occur with other weapons, for which the characteristics of a Gim sword are not presupposed. For example, in the case of choosing a halberd, or *Kwan Do,* the question of whether it is a real weapon or a display one would never be an issue. A functional halberd can weigh four and a half kilos, and, evidently, its blade is rigid and made of good quality steel. However, a version of the same weapon made for its use in exhibitions and tournaments would be made from aluminium and light wood, and its weight would not exceed one and a half kilos. The manufacturing of non-functional display weapons from light materials is something that happens with almost all traditional weapons such as halberds, sabers, or butterfly knives. In any case, training with weapons should always be approached with respect and prudence, as the lightest and flimsiest sword can cause cuts and wounds if used improperly.

THE ORIGIN OF THE FORM

The Yang Style 32-step straight sword Form is a simplified version of the traditional 55-step Form[5]. Still, it presents variations we must carefully observe. Some techniques are different from those of the original Form, and the direction in which certain movements are executed also changes.

The publication of the Form dates back to 1957 as part of an extensive process, undertaken by the Chinese government, aiming to unify the defining criteria of a renewed official martial identity. As a consequence of this publicity effort on the part of the state, sequences such as this one, or the simplified 24-step Form, have enjoyed great expansion throughout the world over the decades. This occurrence, though, also entails some negative aspects. The fact that these are easily accessible routines on many occasions causes their practice to be approached from a self-satisfying point of view, or straight deceiving; to the point where some come to consider fencing as a mere exercise, of an aesthetic or relaxing nature. Without a doubt, practising with the sword can constitute in itself a dynamic Meditation exercise, but only in the case of people educated in the Art of Tai Chi Chuan, and always with sufficient mastery of the technique. Approaching Martial Arts from superficial and simplistic points of view degrades the legacy of generations of Sifus and turns a sublime discipline into a vulgar parody. The Form must be studied for what it is; and, if it is possible, under the tutoring of a qualified instructor familiar with the techniques. In this ideal context, it is normal that discrepancies should be produced between different lineages at the moment of presenting certain aspects of the Form. This technical debate is stimulating and can result enriching; however, differences based on habit or lack of knowledge should be discarded, since they are not endorsed by a prior rigorous analysis.

We must study each technique with care and attention, from the respectful and patient attitude that is inherent to every learning process.

---

5   The traditional straight sword Form of the Yang Tai Chi Chuan is, obviously, the reference sequence within the style for the study of this weapon. Inevitably, the sequence can present some variations depending on the teachings of the different martial lineages. In the same way, the count of the number of techniques that comprise it also differs, it being known as the Form of 51, 54, 55 or 67 steps. In any case, the sequence is, in essence, the same.

FORM

* * *

This third and last section outlines the complete Form illustrated with pictures. To facilitate the comprehension of the different techniques, I have also included snapshots that capture the transitions between movements and the different trajectories of the sword. Moreover, in the final part of this chapter, you can find an appendix with pictures taken from the opposite point of view to that of the complete sequence, in which some details are shown that cannot be seen clearly in the series of pictures that exhibits the whole Form.

When it comes to the enumeration and description of the techniques, I follow the model proposed by Grandmaster Chen Weiming, in his work on the Yang style Tai Chi Chuan straight sword, published for the first time in 1928. Thus, at the bottom of the picture that shows the most representative position of each technique, I have indicated its name, description, and the place it occupies in the sequence. Furthermore, in order to clarify some essential aspects of the Form, the techniques are compared in relation to the empty hand version whenever possible. The description of the techniques does not include explanations about their practical application; since, as previously explained, that level of interpretation necessarily requires the tutoring of a Master.

Regarding orientation, the description of the Form is consistent with the traditional guidelines and it begins on the south-north axis, Yin and Yang[1].

---

1 Literally, dark and bright, is an essential concept of the Taoist thought that has come to be universalised in such a way that it is applied to a variety of fields; from literature to

The series of pictures is divided into four sections that correspond, in turn, to the original segmentation of the Form.

Lastly, it should be pointed out that the translation of some of the techniques that make up the Form varies according to the lineage that records them, in keeping with their own cultural tradition. From an academic point of view, the nomenclature used by Grandmaster Chen Weiming in his work should be taken as a reference, as he was a direct disciple of Grandmaster Yang Chengfu, and the first to publish a book that gathers together the straight sword Form of the Yang style Tai Chi Chuan. Nonetheless, it is very instructive to also pay attention to the different ways of naming the same techniques that other lineages and branches propose, since this allows us to learn from the cultural background that gives them meaning.

---

traditional medicine or even quantum mechanics. In Western culture, it is attributed characteristics that, even though they can facilitate its comprehension, distort its meaning. It is devoid of moral quality, and it does not represent good nor evil. The Taoist perspective of reality is very different from the Hegelian heritage with which the west has built the foundations of its modern philosophical discourse. A good way to come closer to the concept of Yin-Yang is to accept the premise that it is about two extremes of the same concept, opposite and at the same time complementary. Yin and Yang are two polarities that are necessary to establish a virtuous balance, to which the Taoist erudite aspires on his/her path towards illumination.

32 step Yang style
STRAIGHT SWORD FORM

OPENING

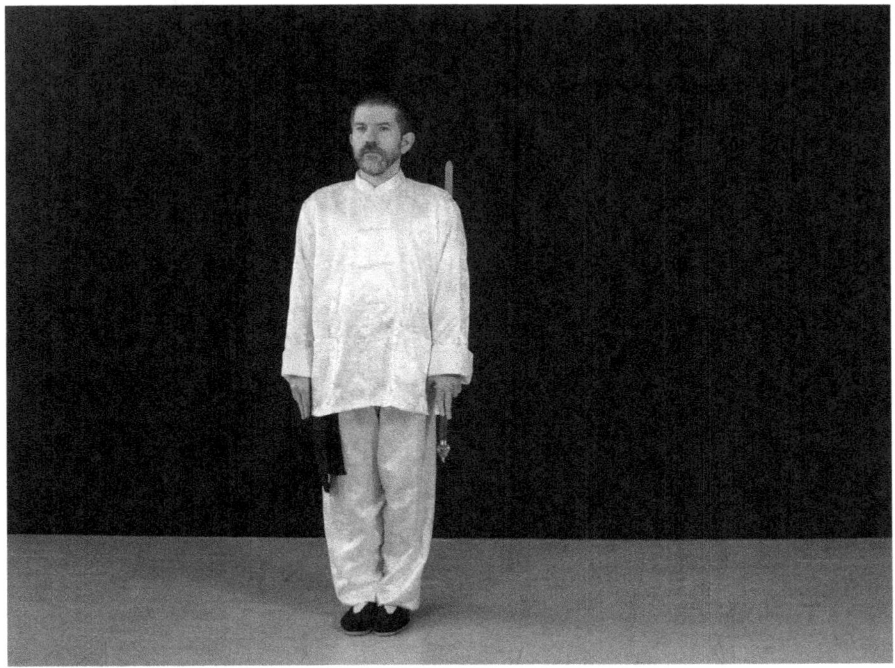

SOUTH. Feet close together and back straight. Hold the sword upside-down with the pommel facing the ground, with your left hand, maintaining the blade flat behind your forearm. The index and middle fingers and the thumb hold the weight of the weapon gripping the guard (*fanwo* position). The right hand forms the secret sword. In this position, *Wu Chi*, firm but relaxed, you can dedicate some minutes to performing a Meditation exercise that will allow you to shut out any distractions and link your Chi to that of the Gim.

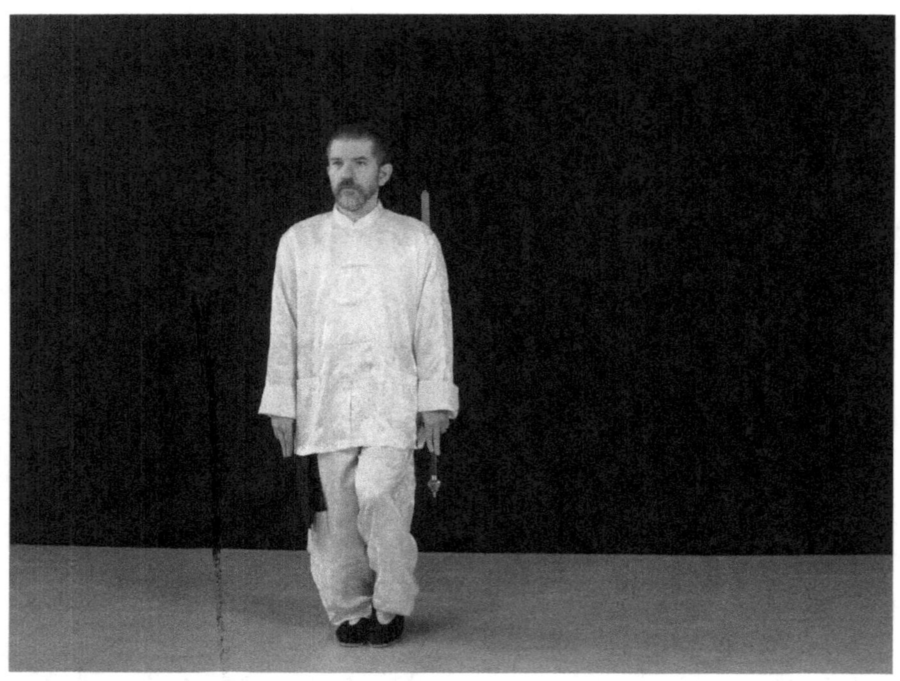

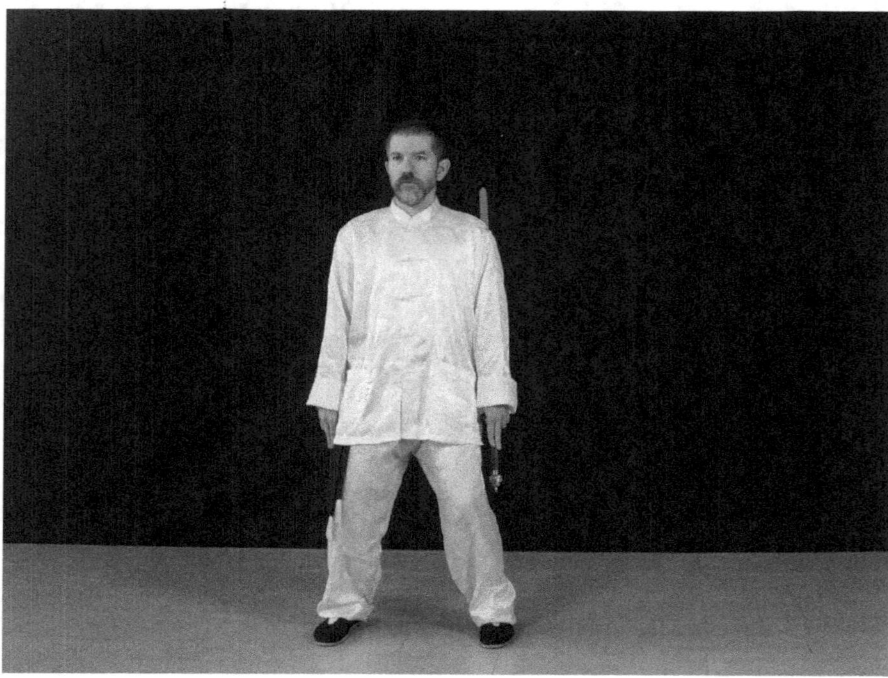

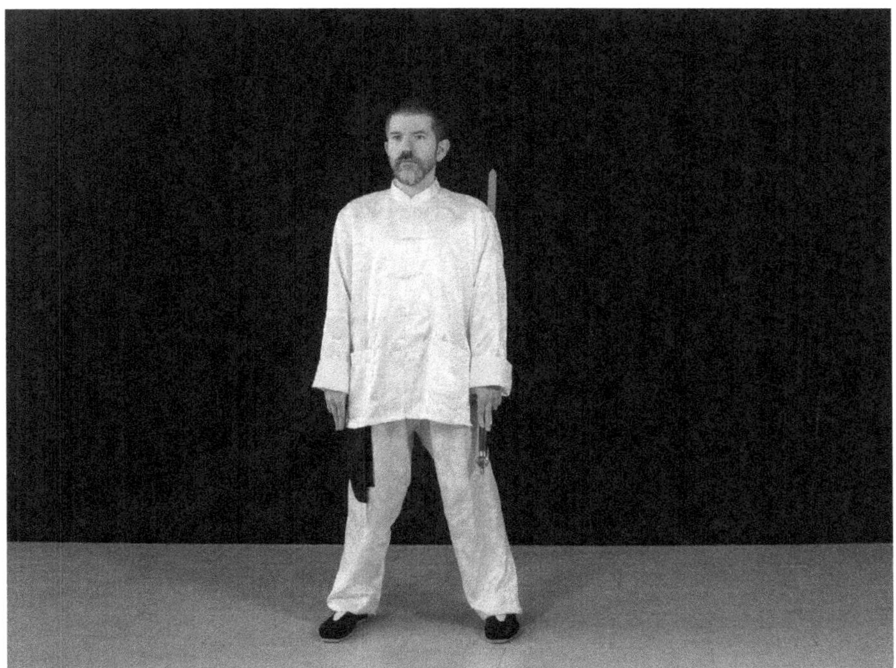

1
Three rings circle the moon - 三環套月

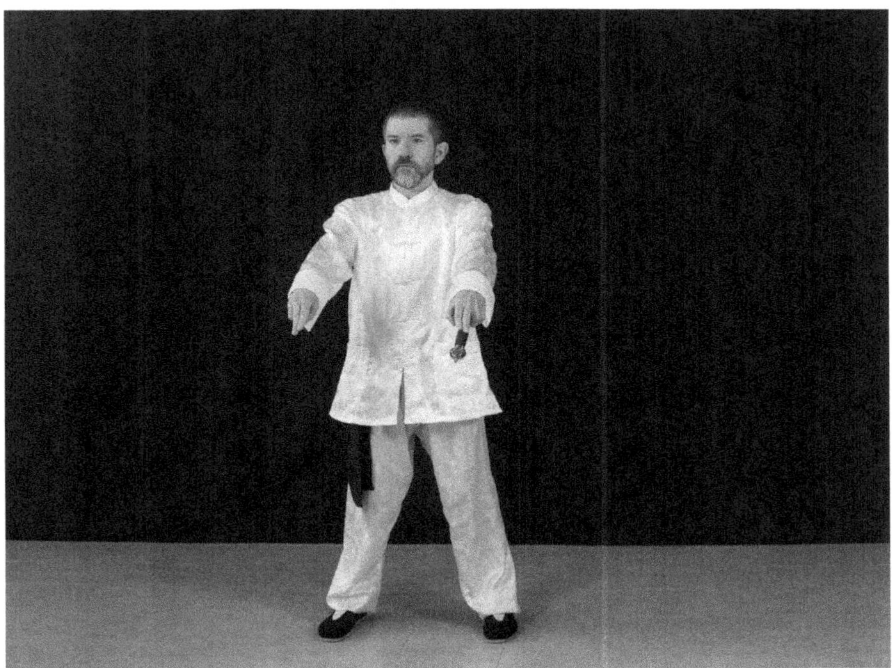

SOUTH. Raise your hands to the height and width of the shoulders. Next, place the weight of your body on your left leg to allow the correction of the right foot toes and the rotation of the torso and waist to the east, direction in which the technique is concluded. The left arm, with the elbow bent, holds the sword. The right hand prepares to continue the movement from the height of the temple. This technique, known, among other names, as *The immortal shows the way*, is similar to *Brush knee.*

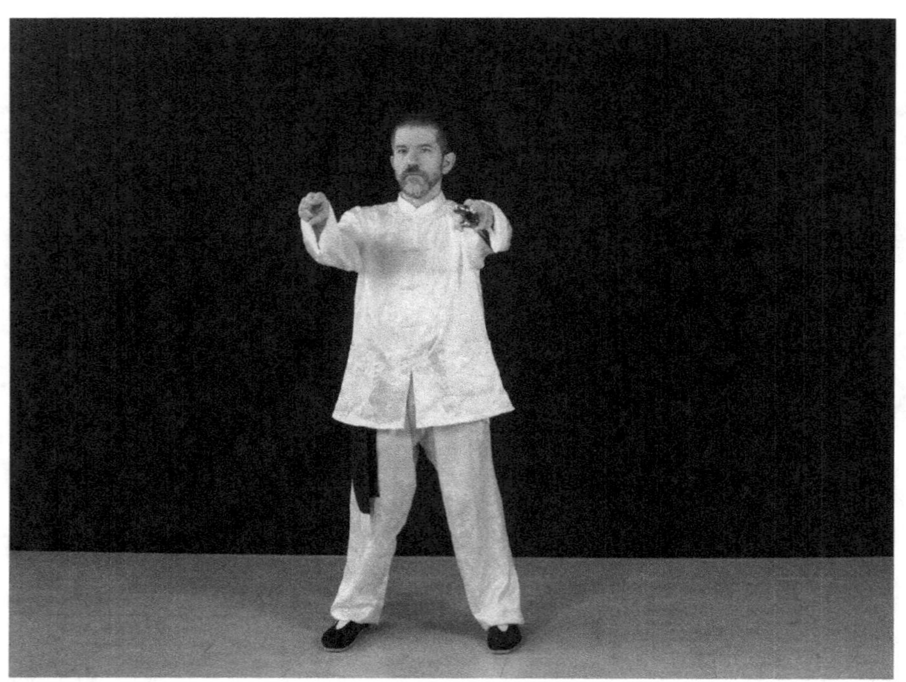

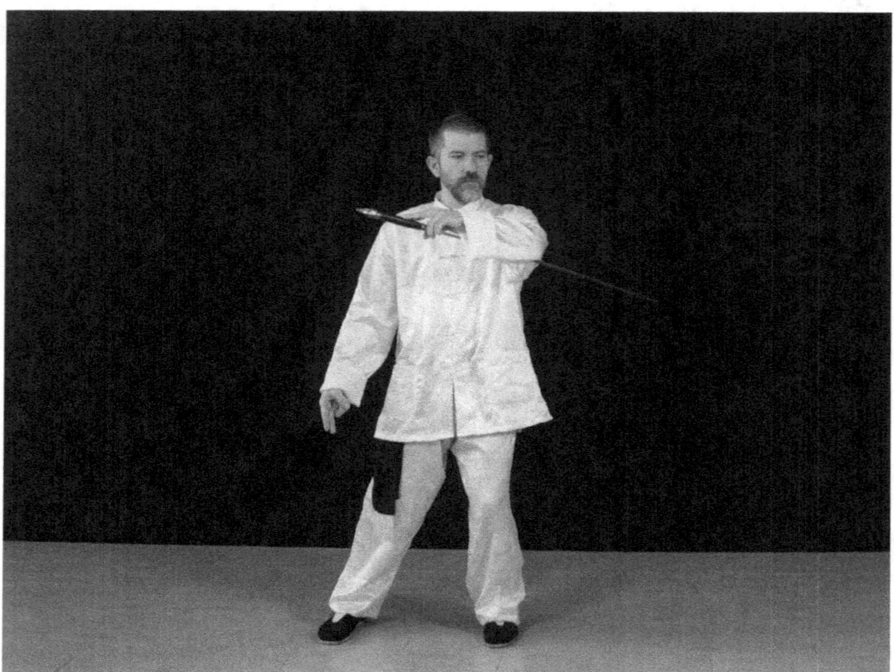

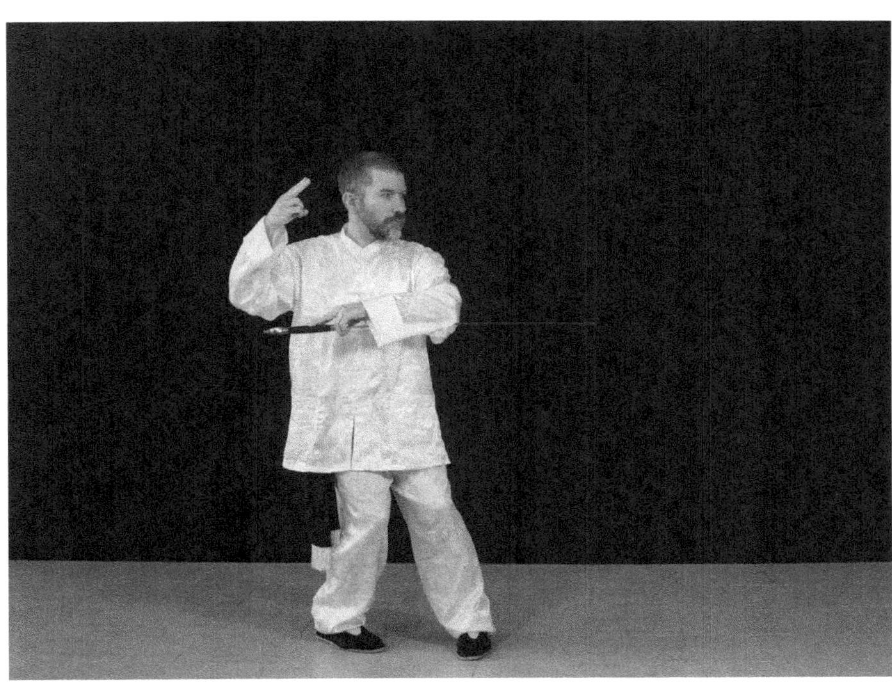

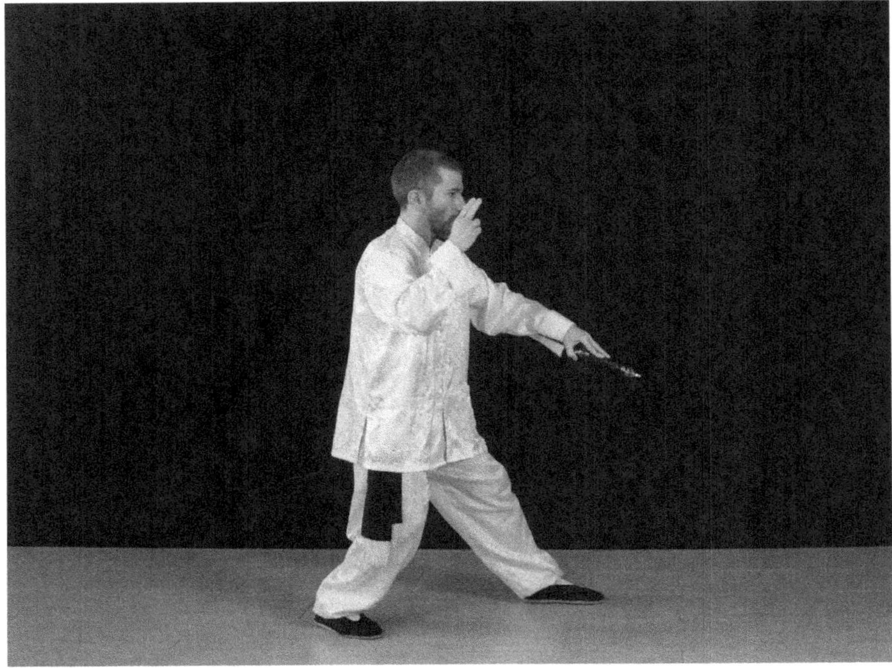

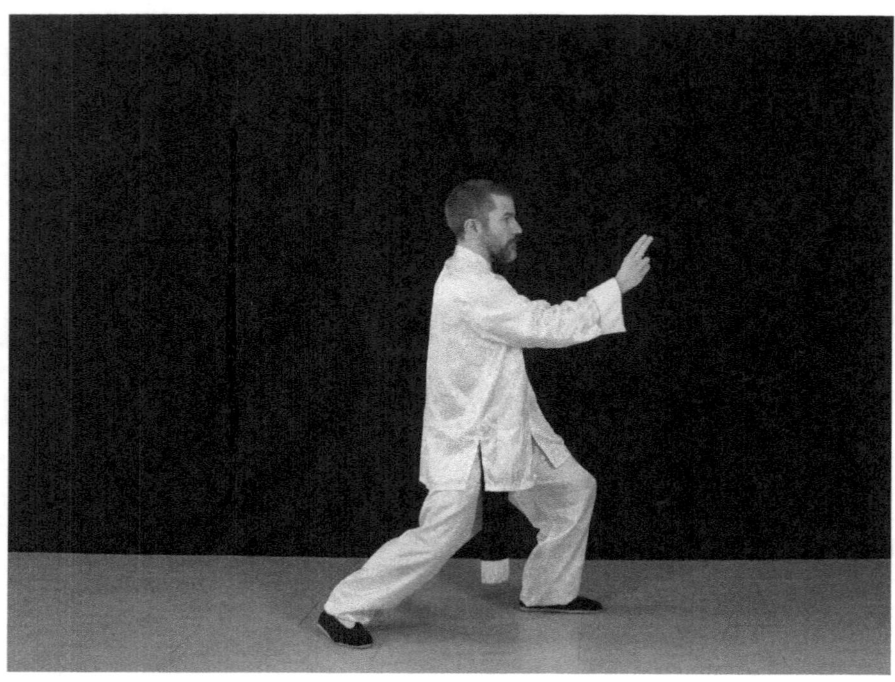

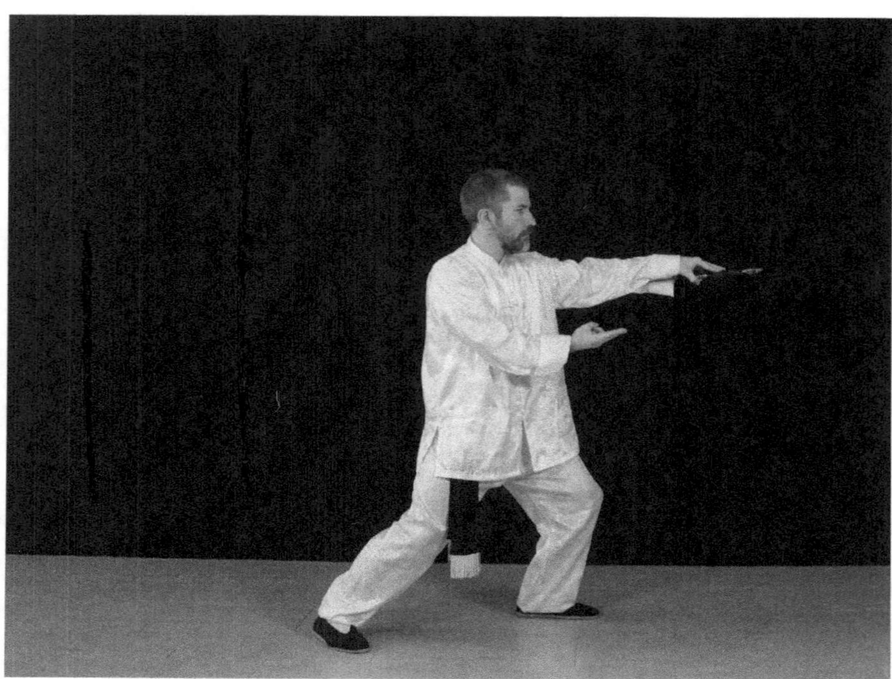

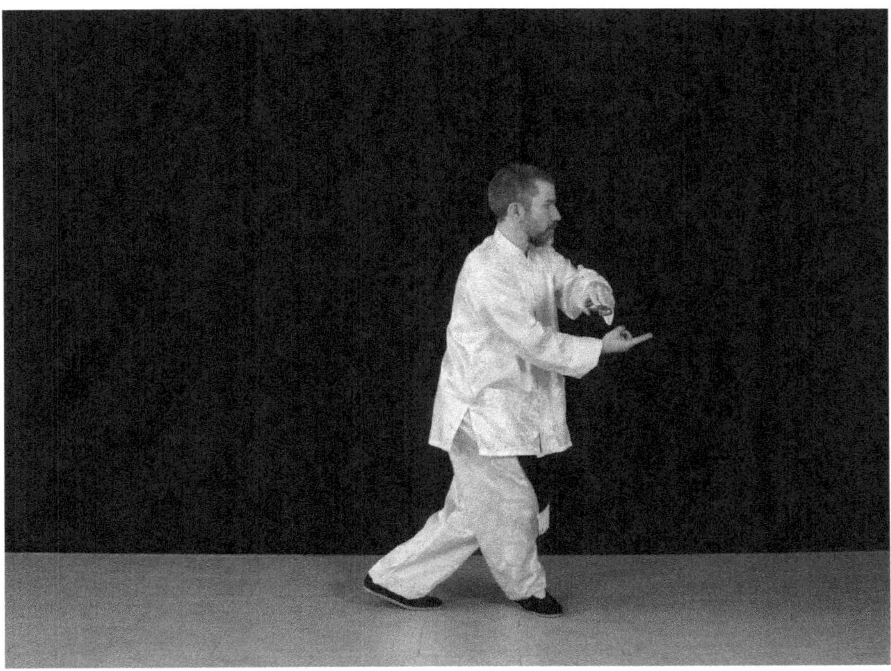

EAST. Step forward crossing your right foot in front of the left one in the way of quai ma. Extend both arms keeping the hands approximately at the height of the shoulders. The secret sword points to the west, maintaining the bottom part of the right wrist facing up. The left hand holds the sword, perpendicular to the ground (*zhimian*).

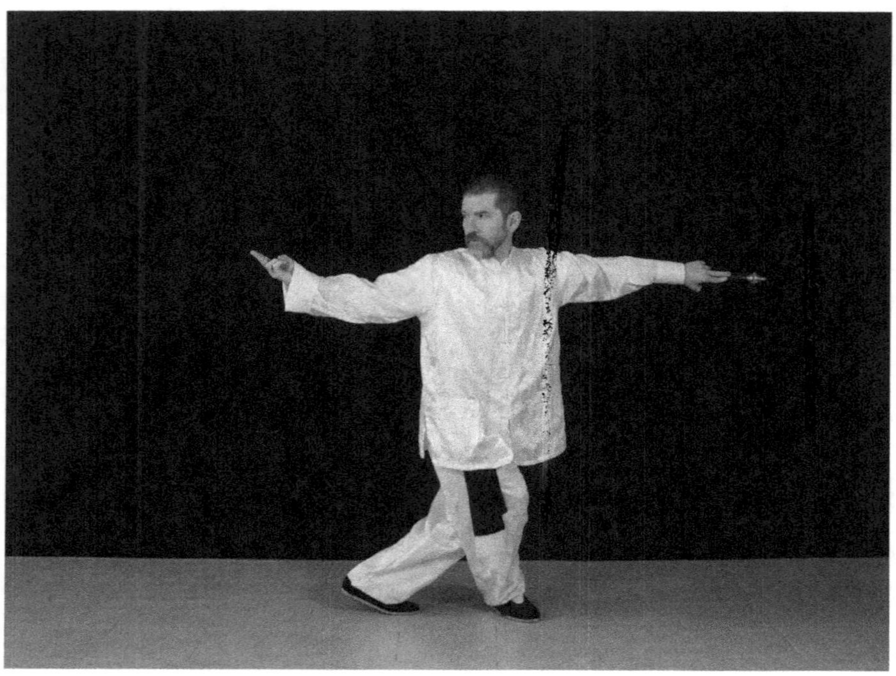

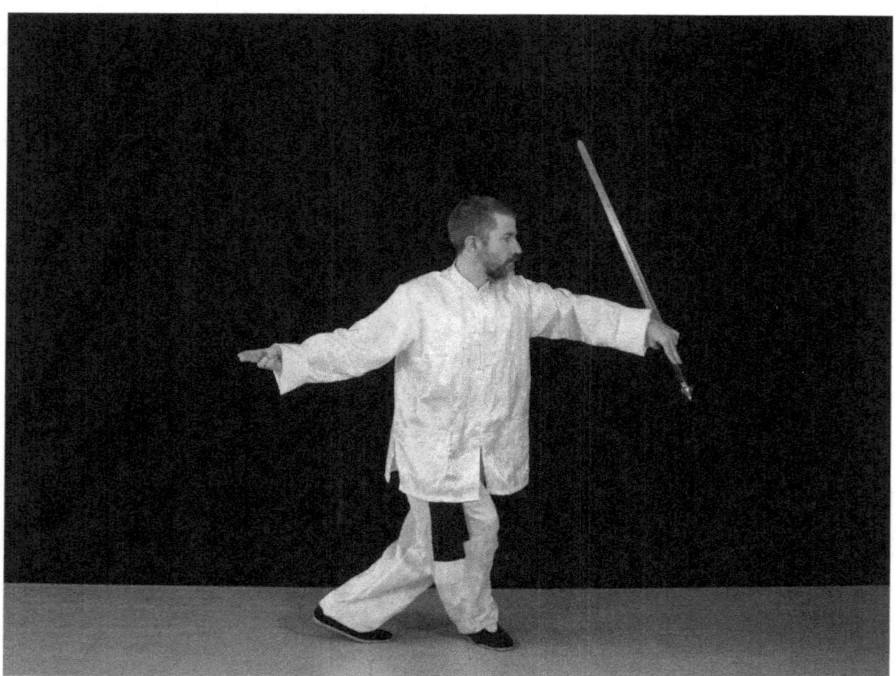

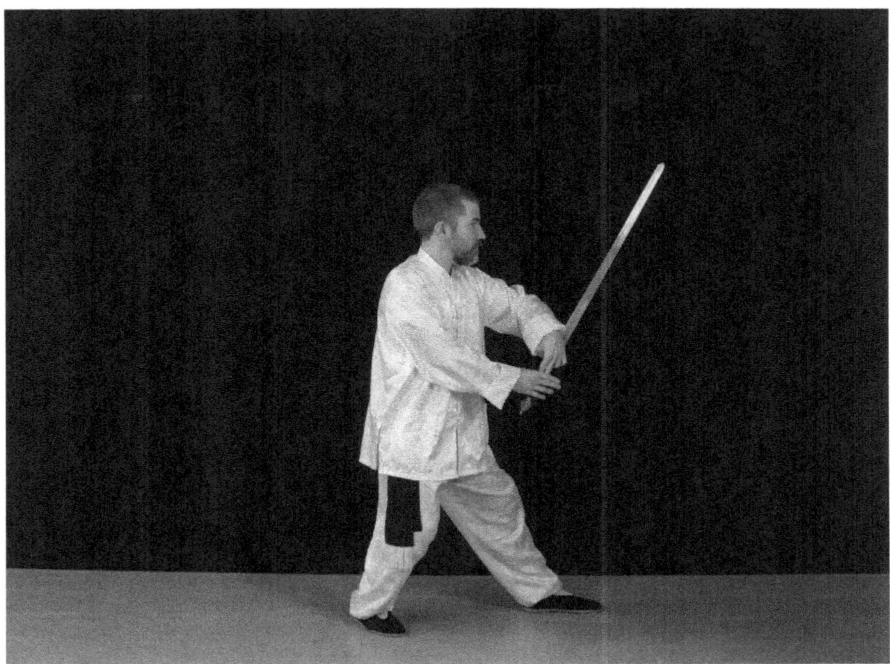

EAST. Advance with the left foot. Take a step with the right foot to bring both feet together, keeping the knees bent. Turn the sword clockwise to separate it from the forearm. After relaxing the grip, the right hand wields the sword and continues with the circular trajectory of the movement. The tip of the sword ends its route pointing east, slightly tilted to the ground.

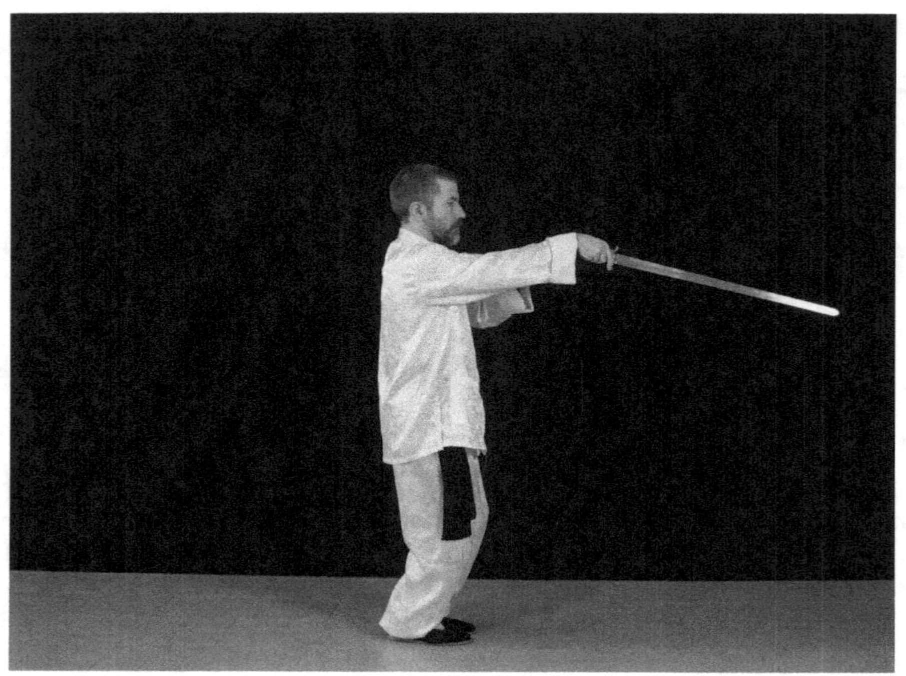

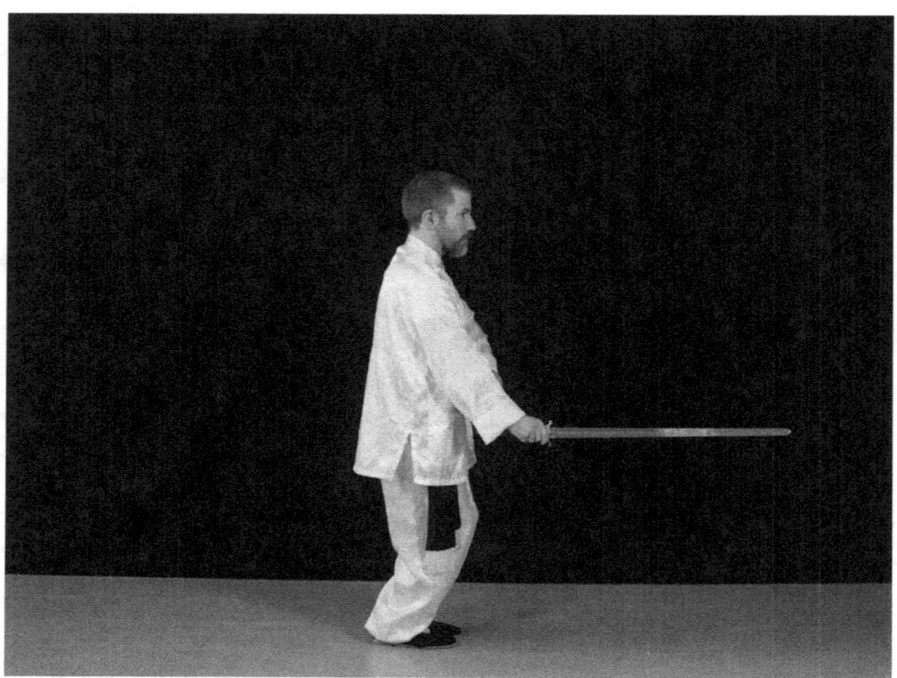

2
The great star of the Literary God - 魁星势

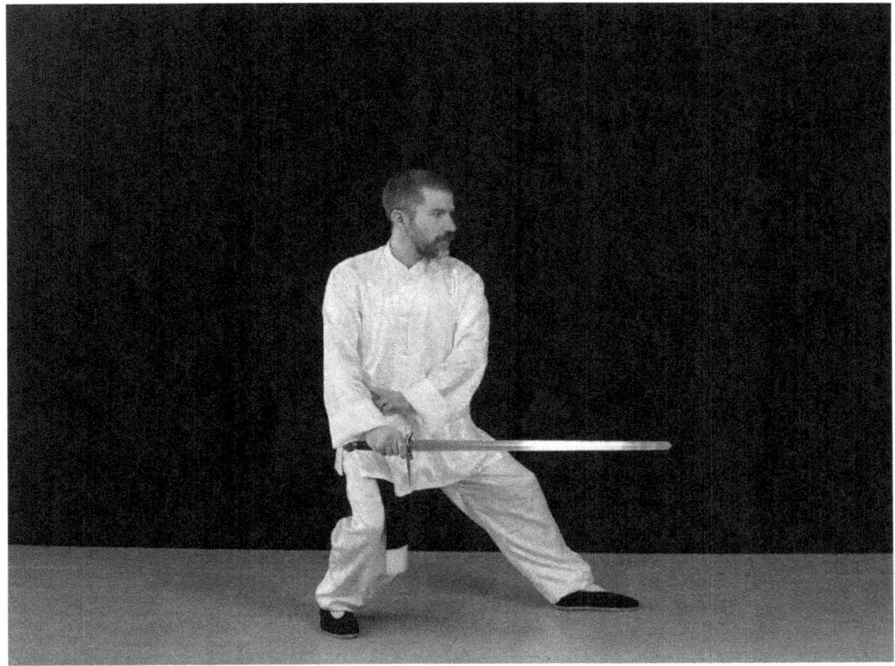

EAST. Lower the right wrist to the level of the tip of the Gim. Step back with your right leg into an extended bow stance. Placing the weight of the body on the right leg, pull the sword. After that, the blade describes a wide arc southeast, and the point ends up facing the sky at a forty-five-degree angle. The eyes follow the point of the sword. Rotate your waist to the right.

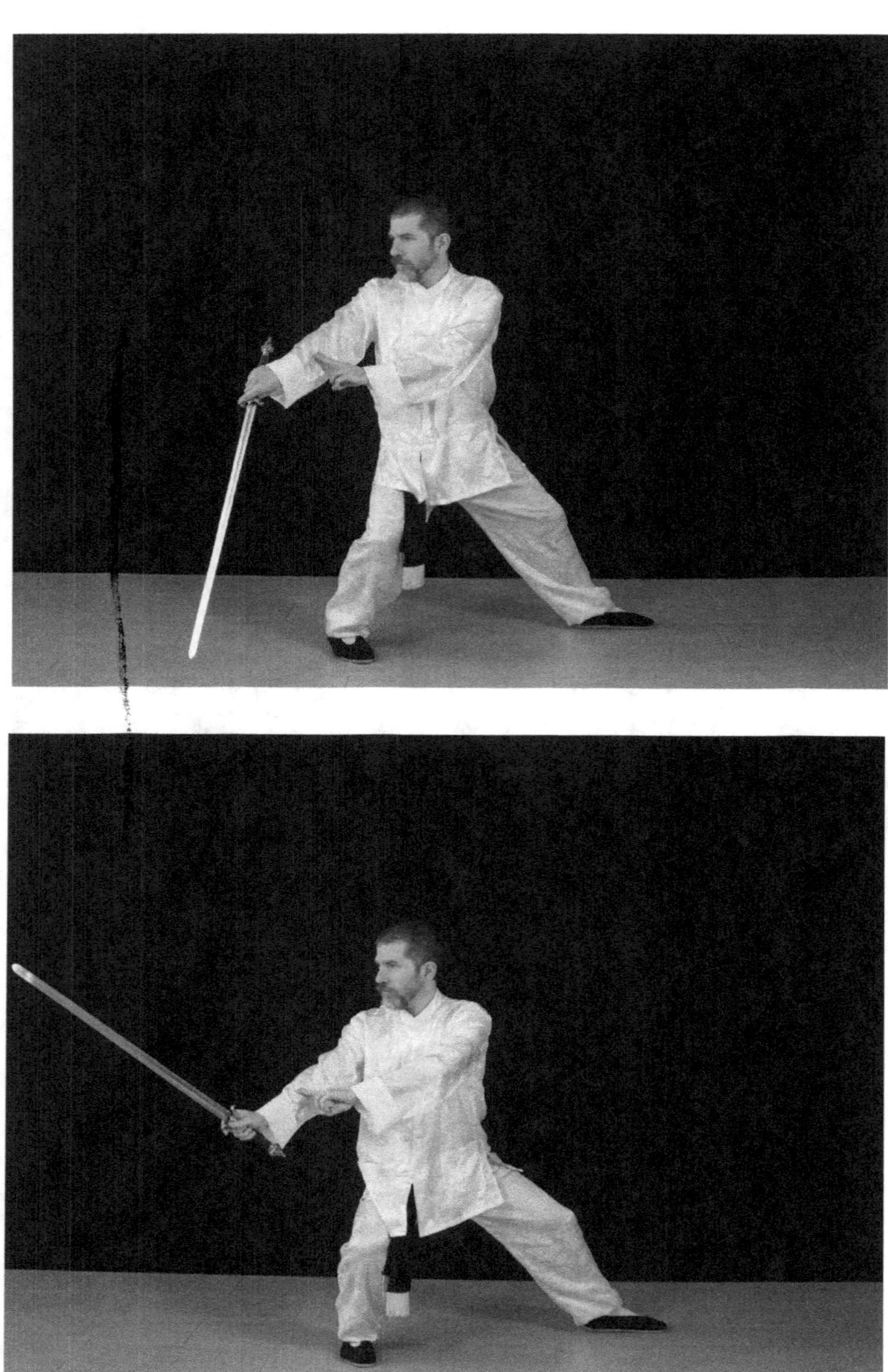

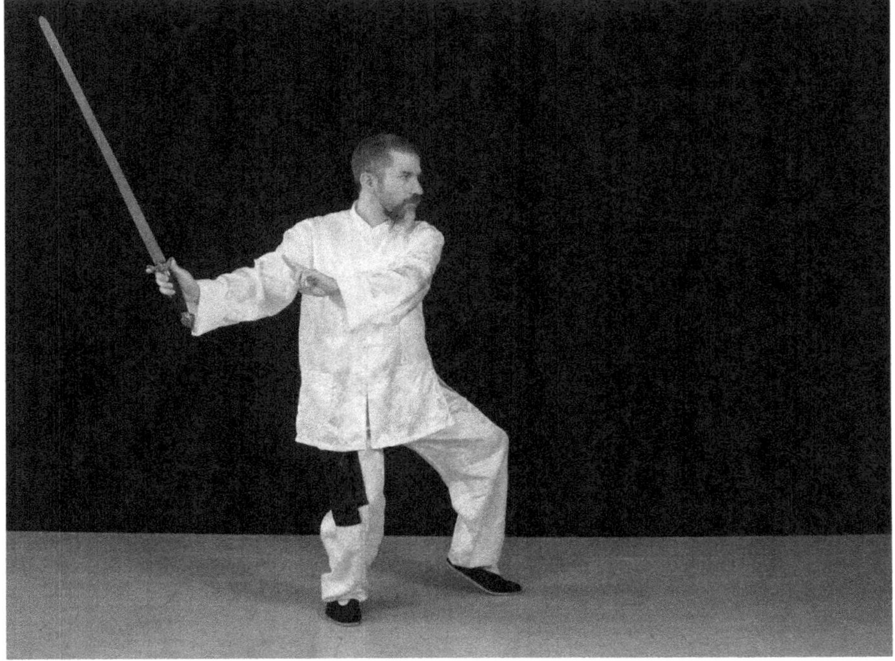

Carrying on, the sword follows its natural trajectory until it comes back to the east, and the left leg comes back into the middle step of the bow stance. The waist turns towards the centre.

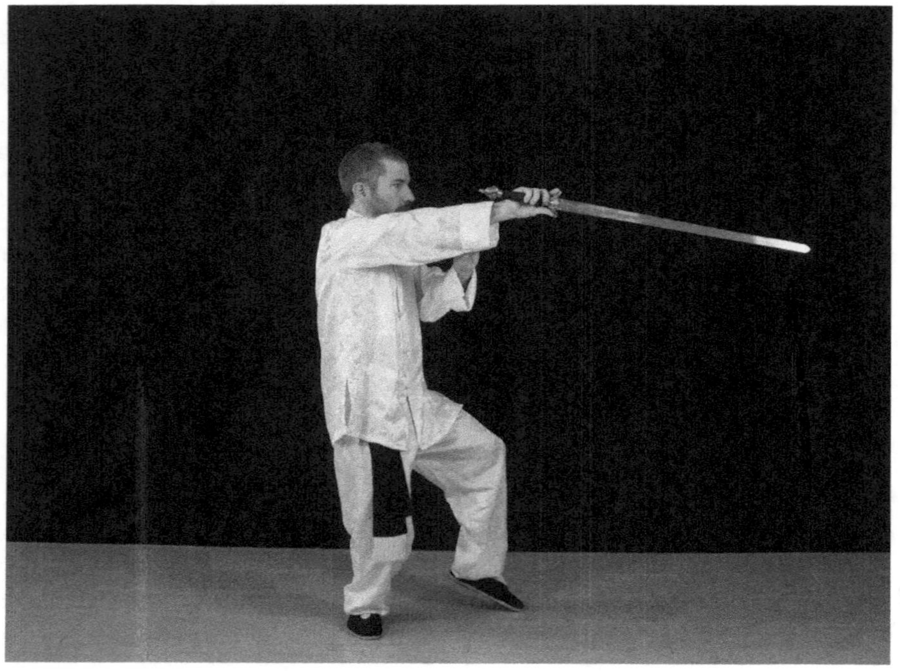

Finally, the sword is placed above the head, perpendicular to the ground, and the left foot is lifted as in *The golden rooster rests on one leg*. The secret sword points east.

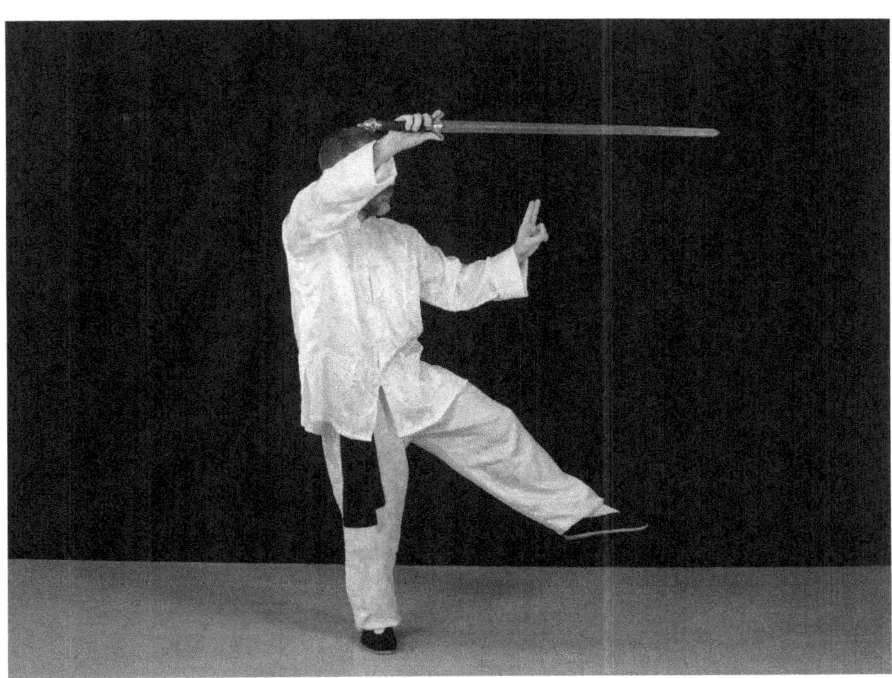

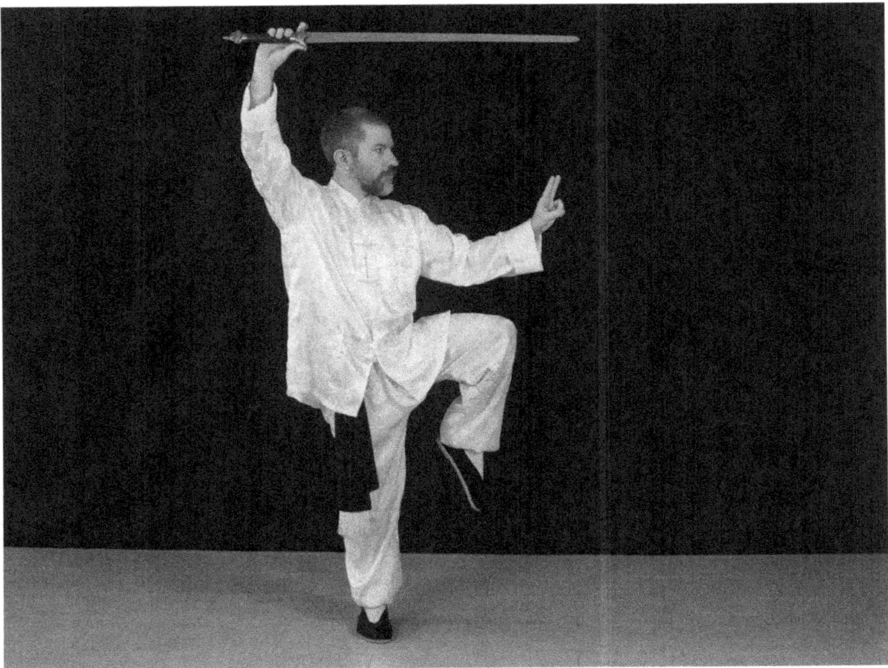

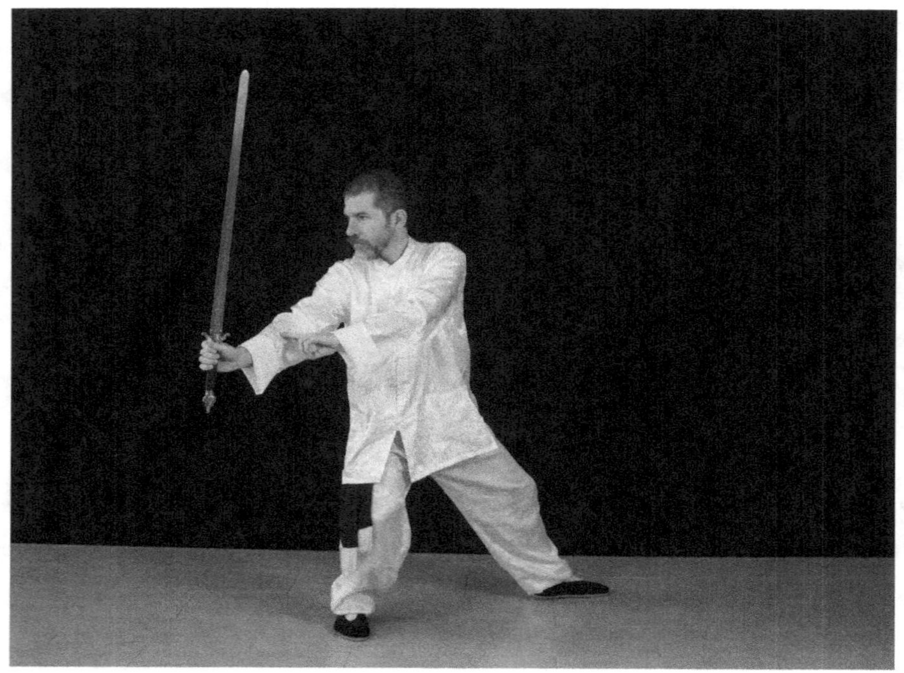

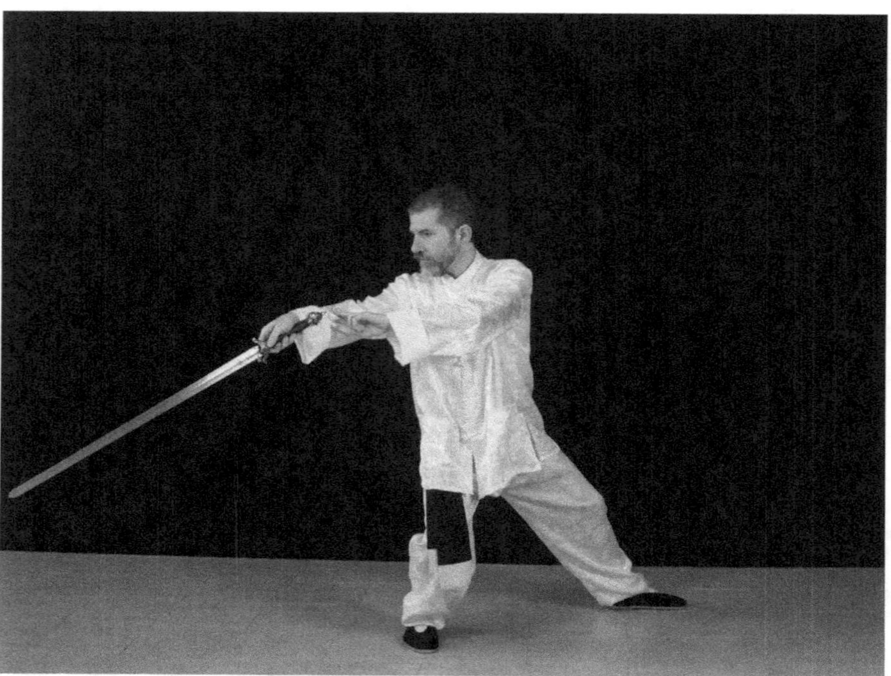

3
The swallow dips its beak in the water - 燕子抄水

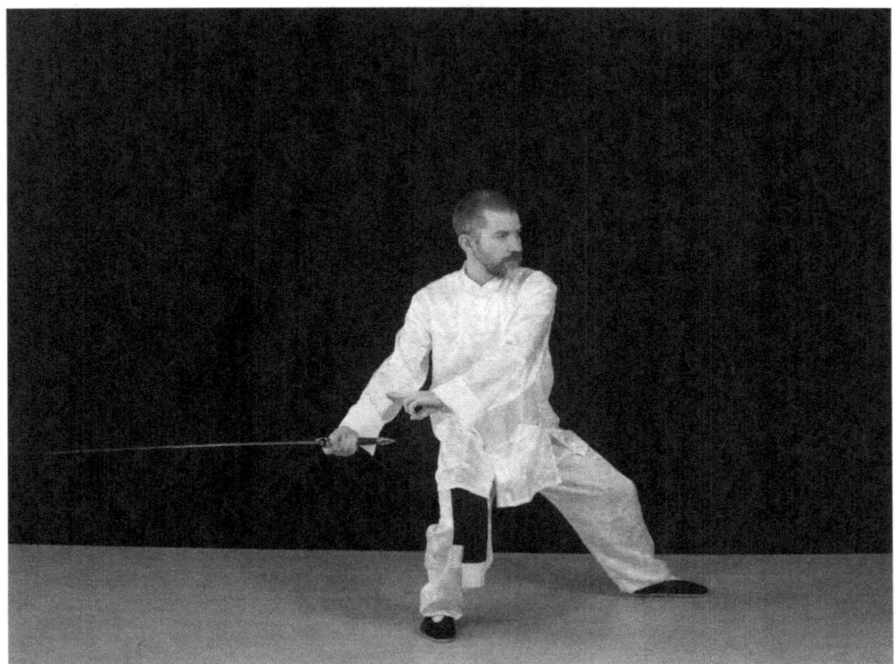

EAST. Place the sword in pingmian position. During the shift of the weight that has the objective of getting you into the bow stance, the sword describes an ample circular cut towards the east followed by the turn of the waist. The point of the sword should be oriented slightly towards the northeast at the end of the movement. The left hand remains above the head, on the left flank, with the back towards the forehead. This technique bears a resemblance to *The fair lady works the shuttle*.

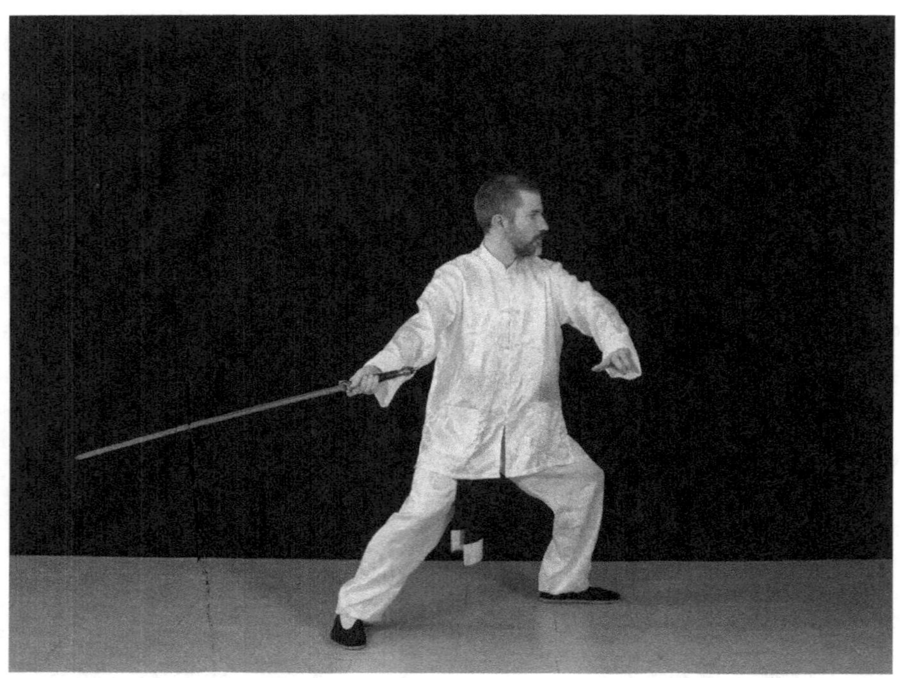

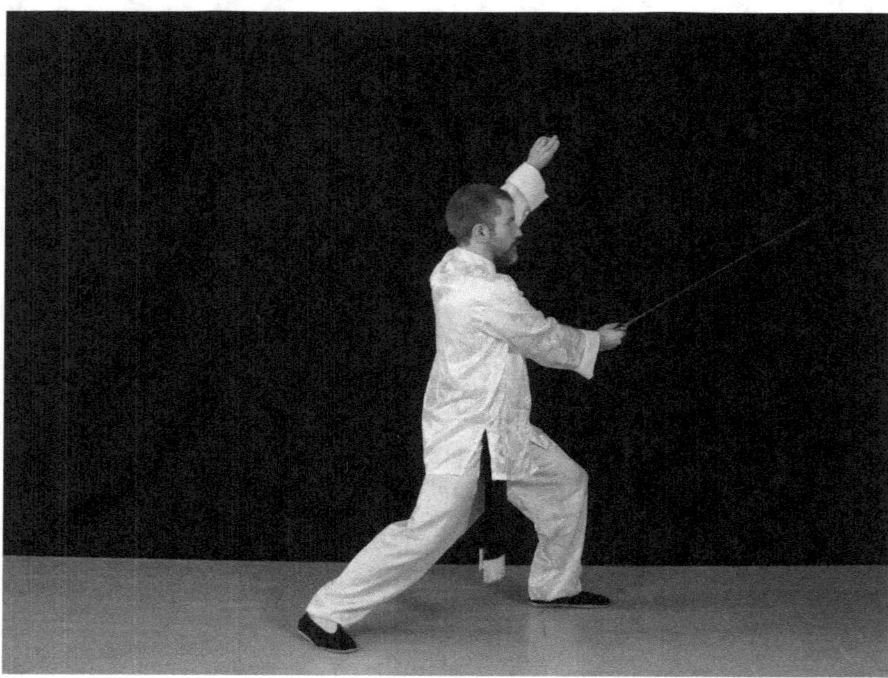

4
Block and sweep to the right - 右边拦扫

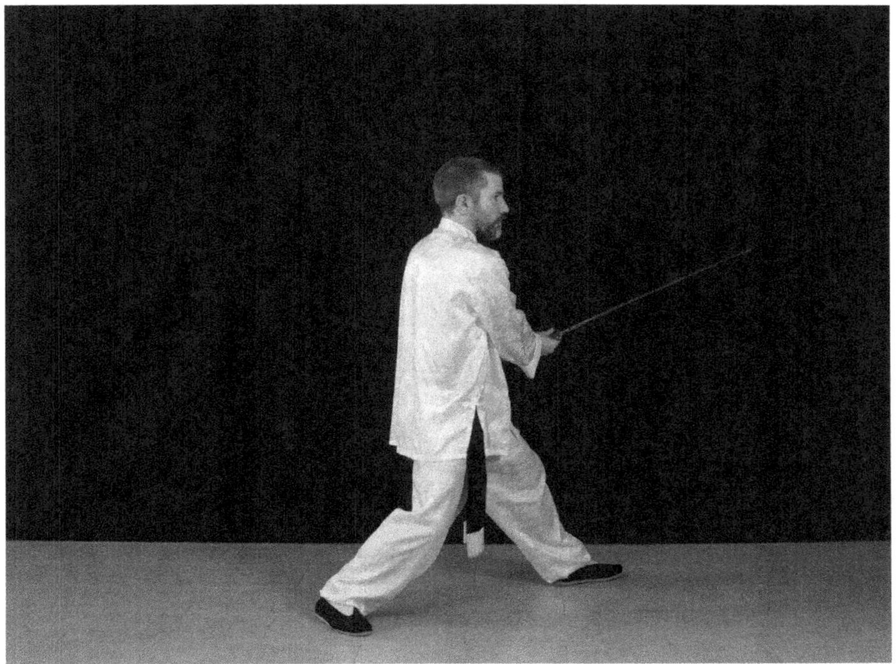

ESTE. Step forward into the right bow stance. The right wrist turns one hundred and eighty degrees to the left, and the secret sword rests on the right forearm. Perform a cut to the southeast turning the waist in the same direction. The point of the sword should remain more centred than in the previous technique. In the work of Chen Weiming, this technique is also related to *The fair lady the shuttle*.

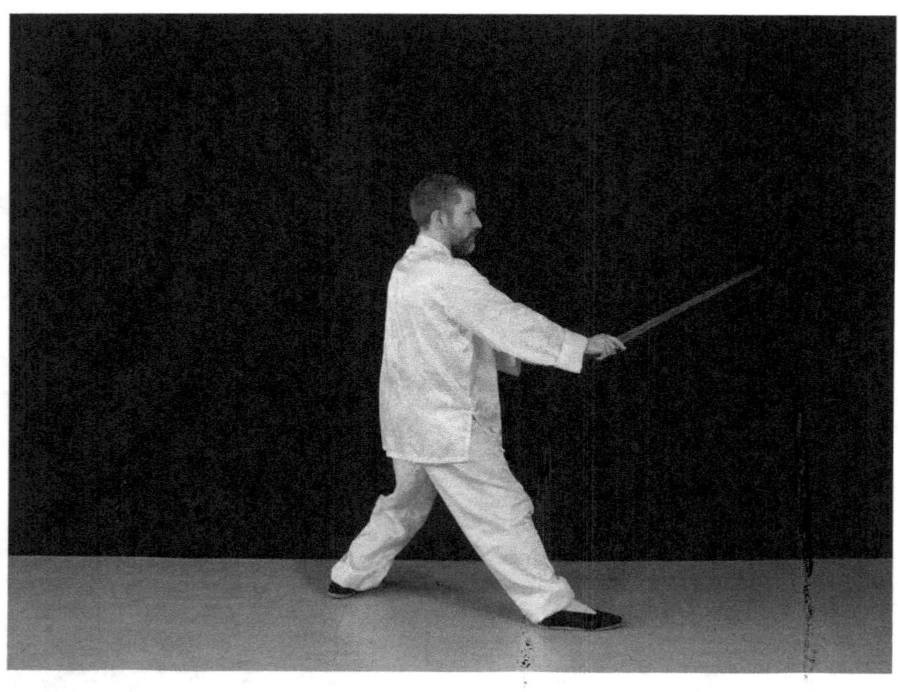

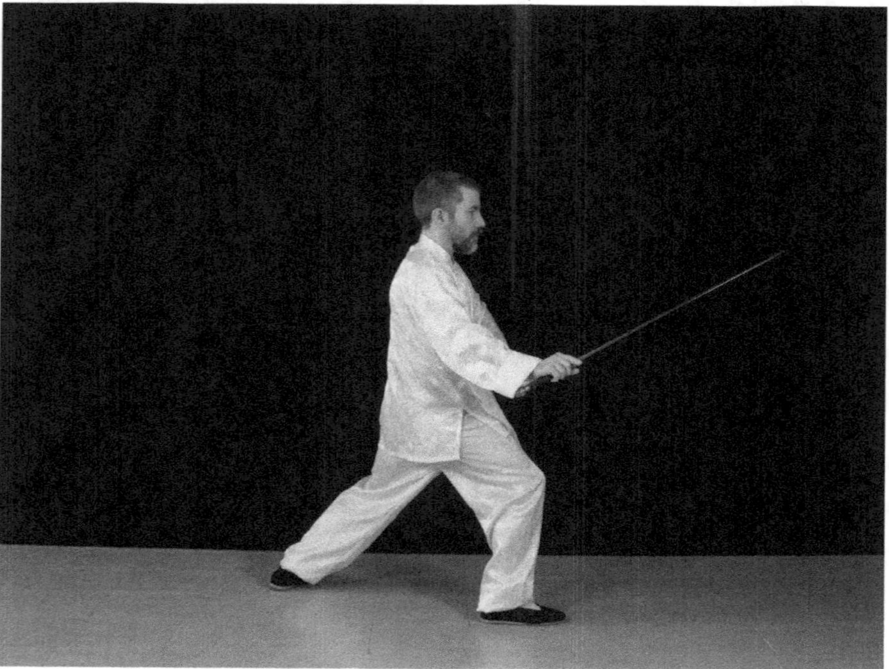

5
Block and sweep to the left - 左边拦扫

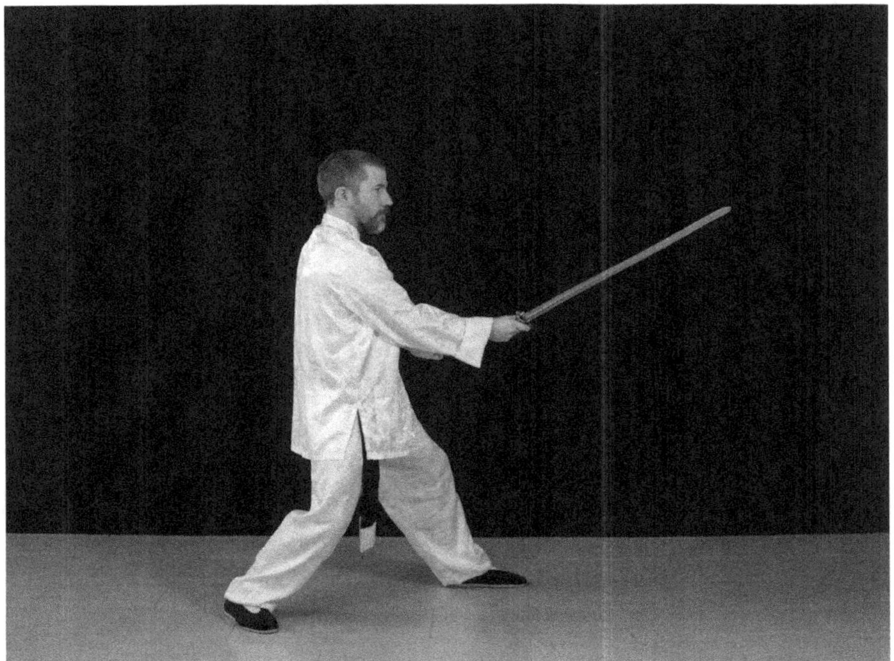

EAST. It is the same technique, but stepping forward into the symmetrical bow stance. The left hand is separated from the forearm and is placed on the left flank in front of the head. The waist returns to the centre.

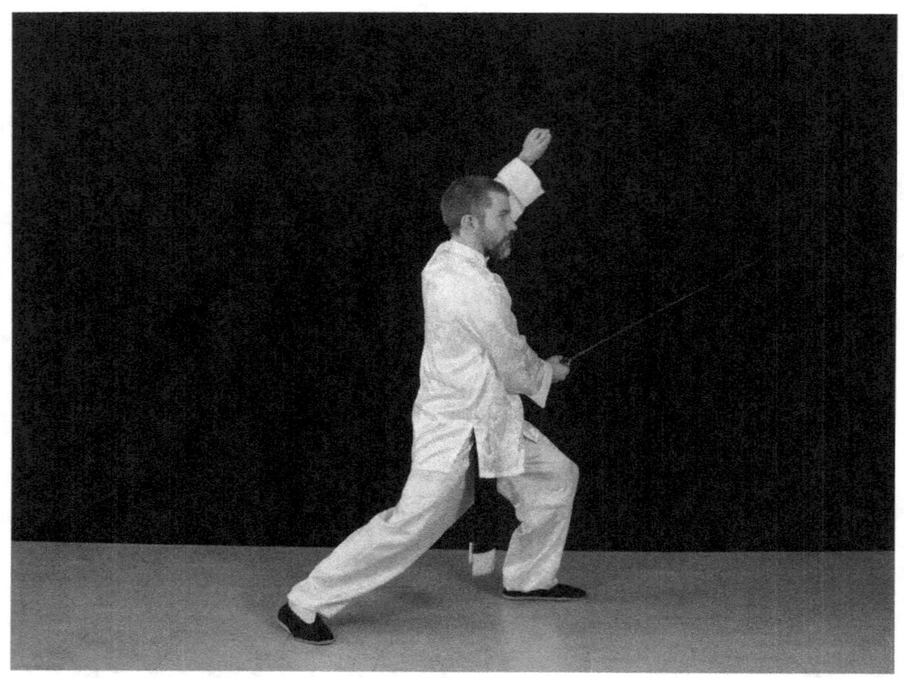

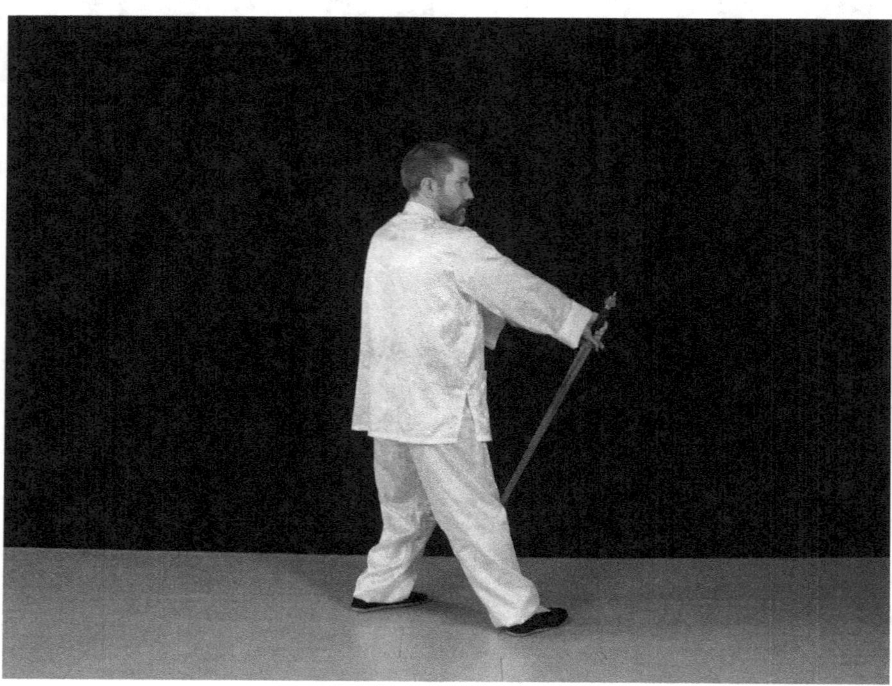

6
The night demons explore the sea - 夜叉探海

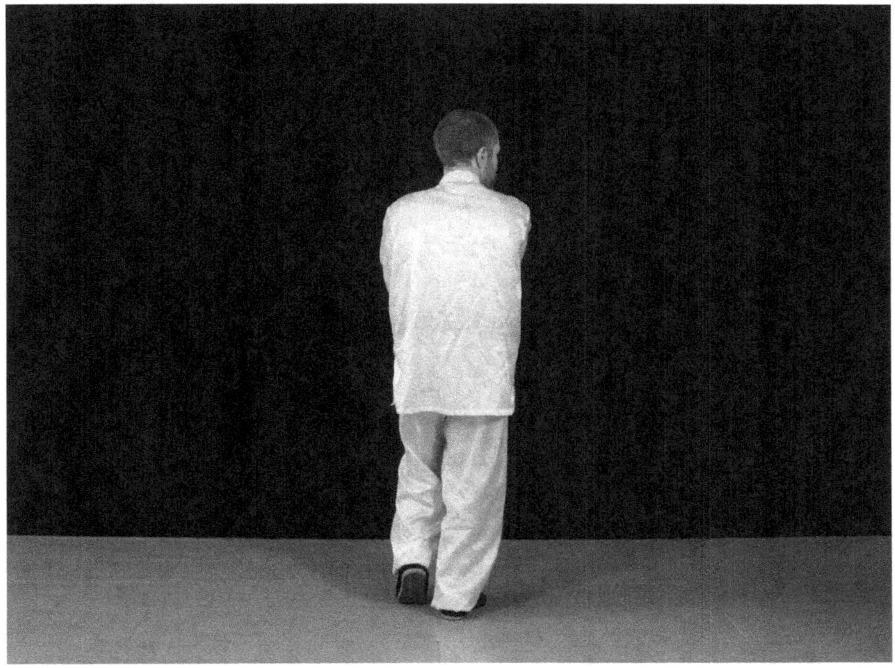

EAST. Advance with the right leg, placing the toes so that they face north. Most of the body weight rests on your right leg. The left foot is placed behind the right one, parallelly, with the heel lifted.

Turn the torso orienting it towards the right foot toes, in such a way that your right shoulder remains towards the north. At the same time, place the sword in front of your abdomen with the tip facing the ground. The index and middle fingers of the left hand are placed on the right forearm. From this static position, the right wrist turns clockwise until the tip of the sword points downwards at a forty-five-degree angle in terms of the ground. At that point, turn your right wrist one hundred and eighty degrees to execute a straight thrust. The left leg is lifted, maintaining the toes of the left foot facing down. The secret sword rises above the head.

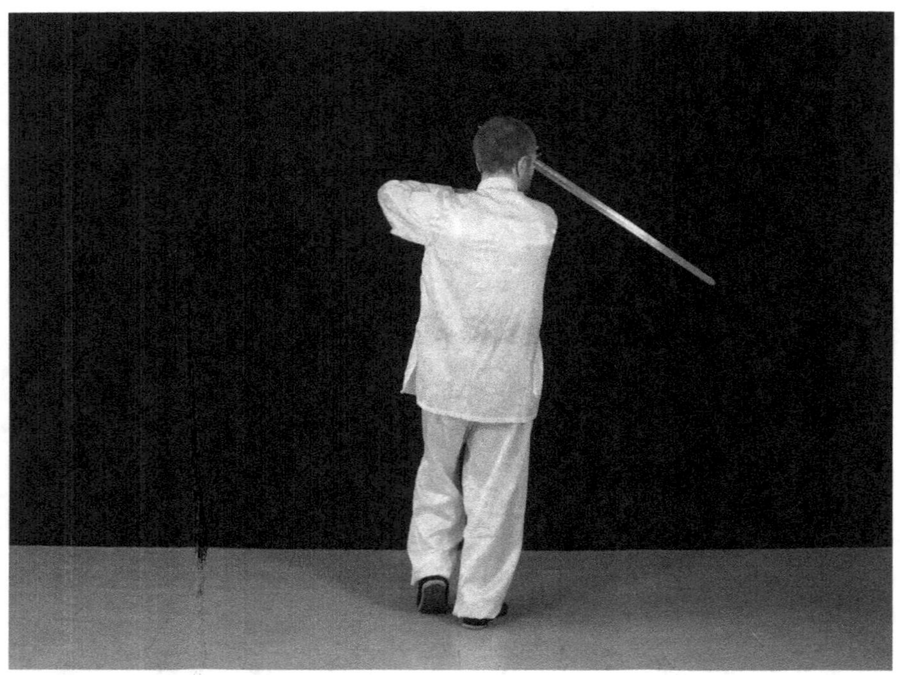

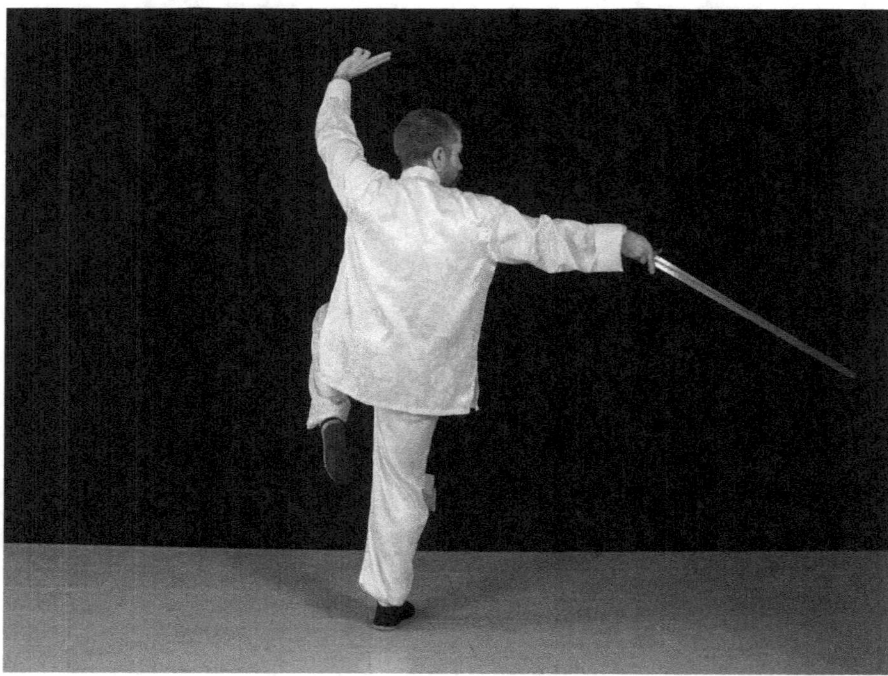

7
Clasping the moon to the bosom - 懷中抱月

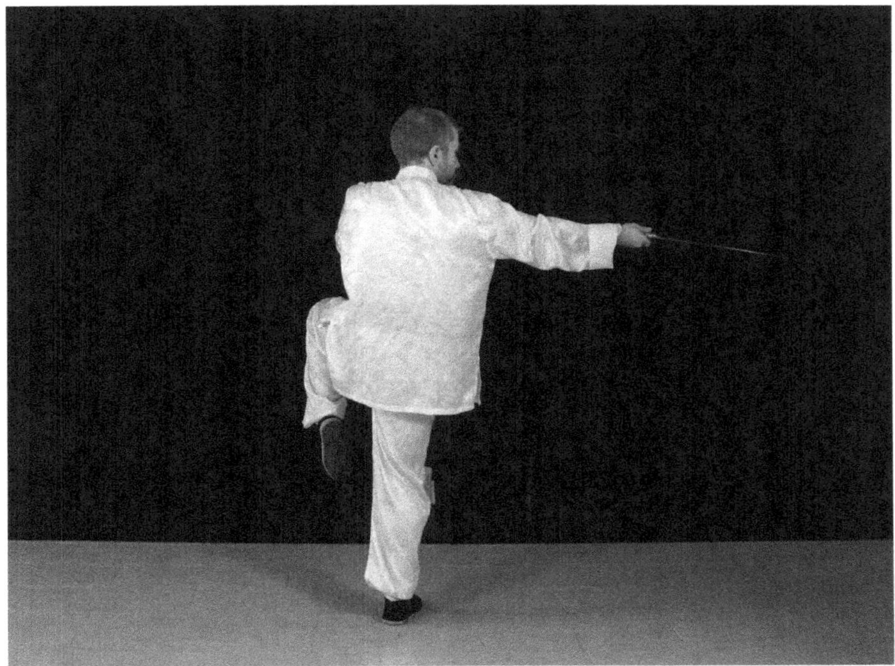

EAST. Place the sword in *pingmian*. The index and middle fingers of the left hand are placed on the pommel. From the previous position, step back into the middle step of the bow stance with your left foot, with the torso facing east.

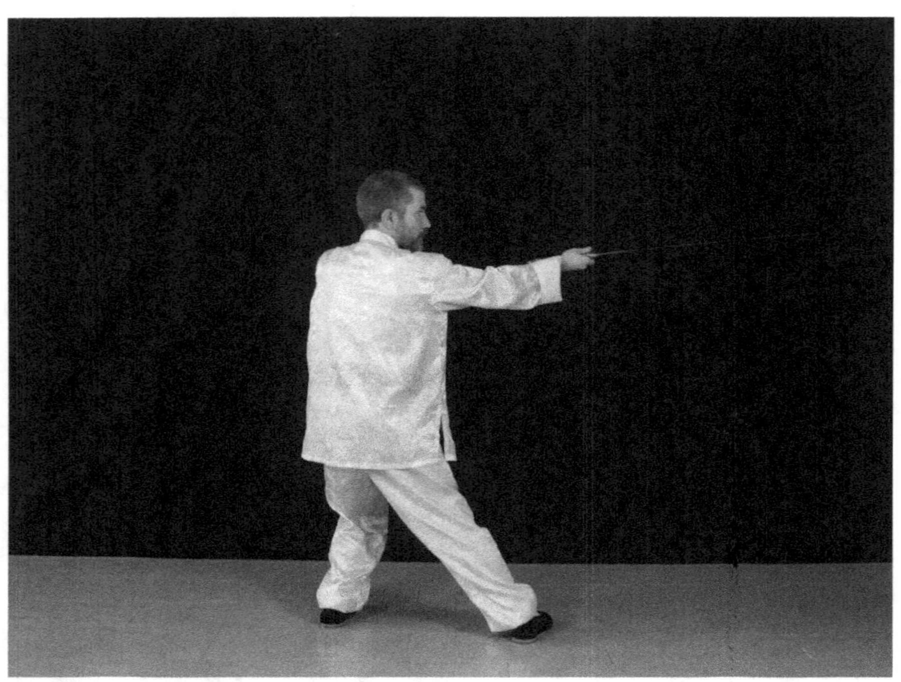

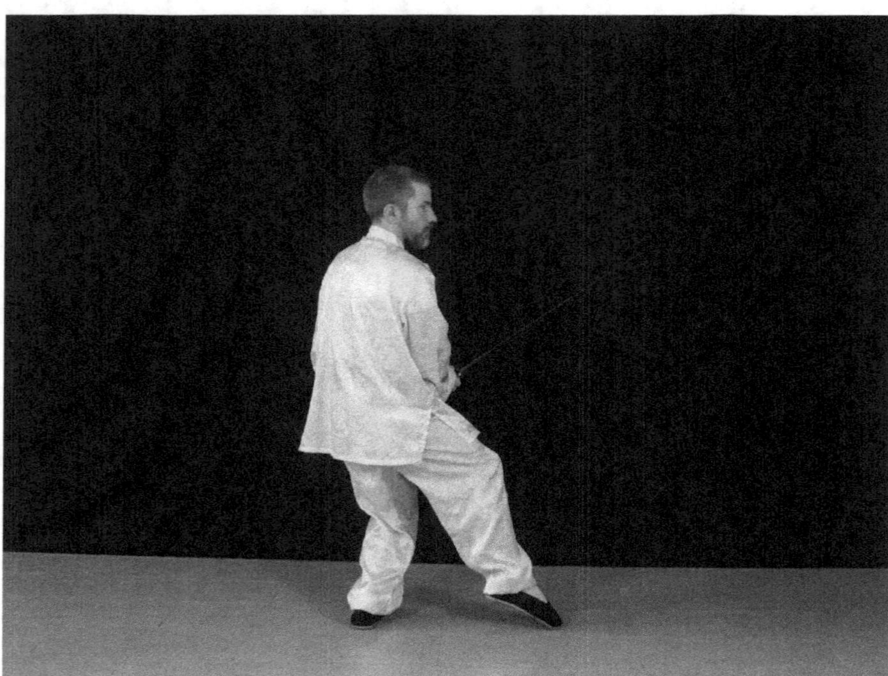

8
The sleeping birds return to the forest - 宿鳥投林

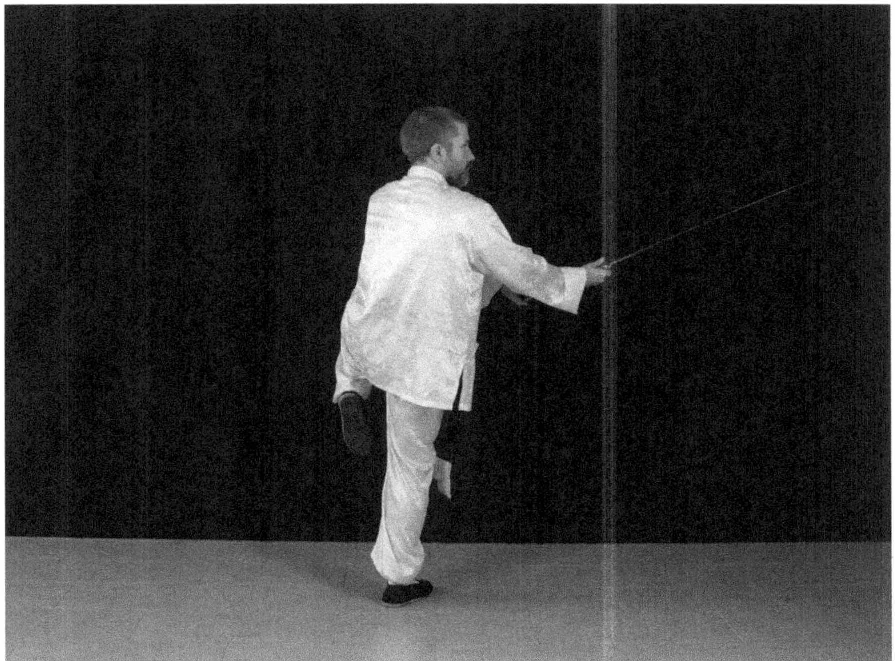

EAST. From the middle step of the bow stance, you should reproduce the position of technique number 6, slightly modifying the placement of the left leg to maintain the balance. In this case, the sole of your left foot must remain parallel to your right leg. Lastly, raise the tip of the sword towards the east, maintaining a forty-five-degree angle with the ground. The trajectory of the movement of the sword should not be rectilinear, but slightly curved.

SECOND SECTION

9
The black dragon whips its tail - 烏龍擺尾

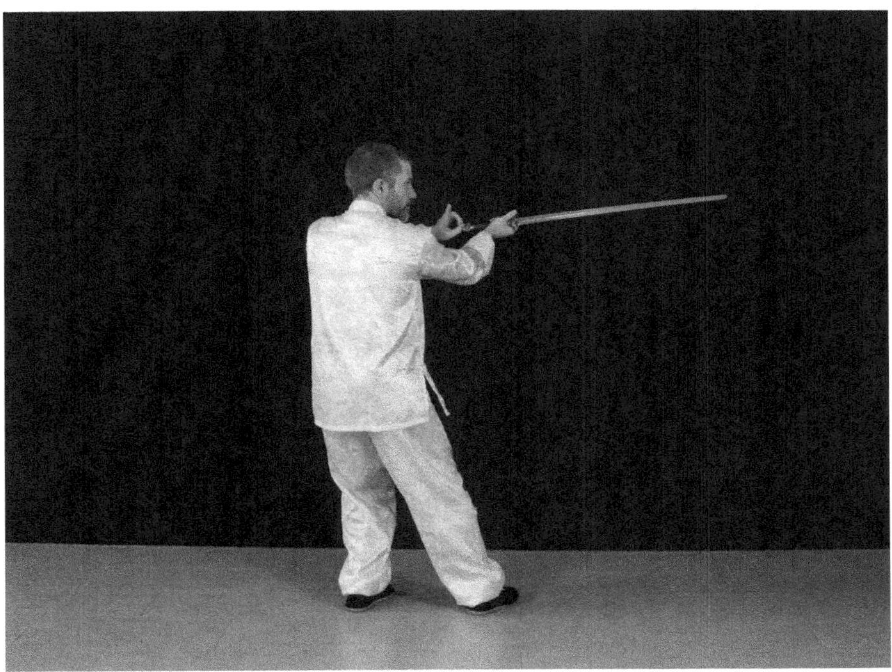

EAST. Rest the left foot on the ground to get into the middle step of the bow stance. The body weight rests mostly on your left leg. Pick up the sword describing an anti-clockwise descending arc, turning the wrist so that the sword blade assumes a vertical position, or *zhimian*. The right arm passes in front of the left one completing the trajectory of the cut that ends in front of your right knee, with the point of the sword towards the ground, in a southeast direction, slightly tilted. During the execution of the technique, the waist turns to the left and comes back to the centre. The secret sword ends up on the left flank above the head. This technique reminds us of *The white crane spreads its wings*, but inverting the position of the arms.

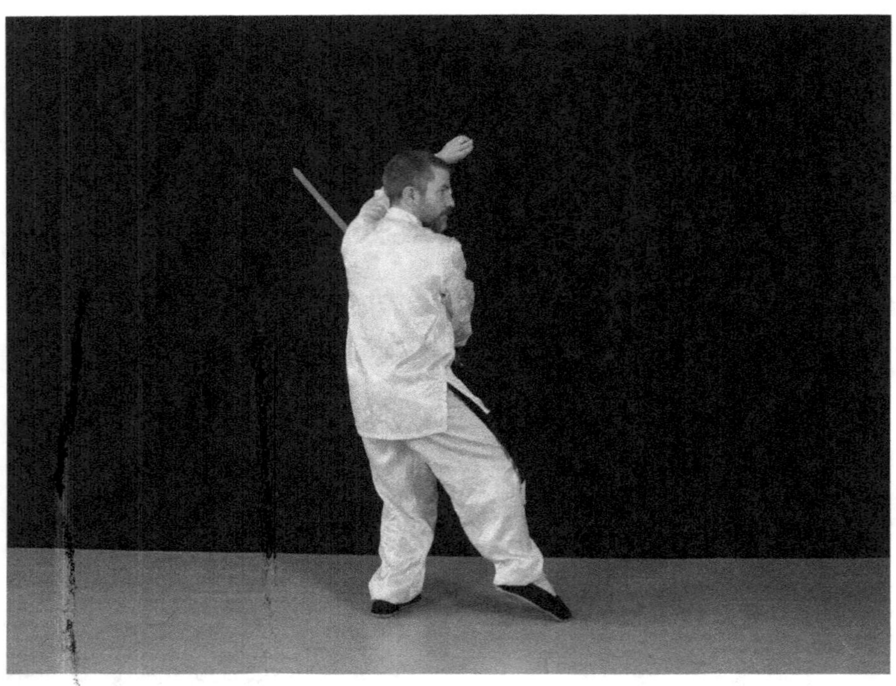

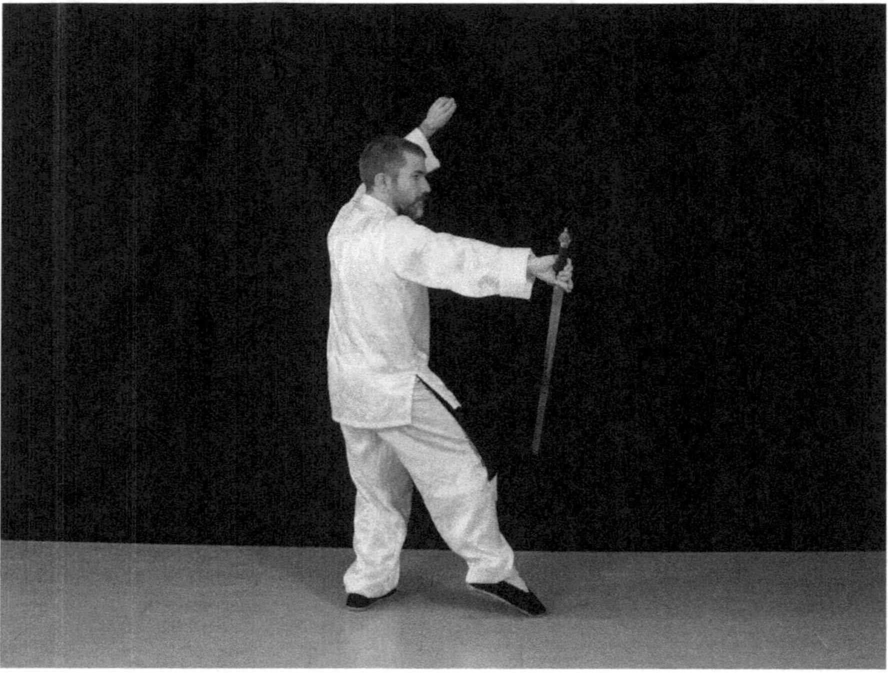

10
The green dragon emerges from the water - 烏龍擺尾

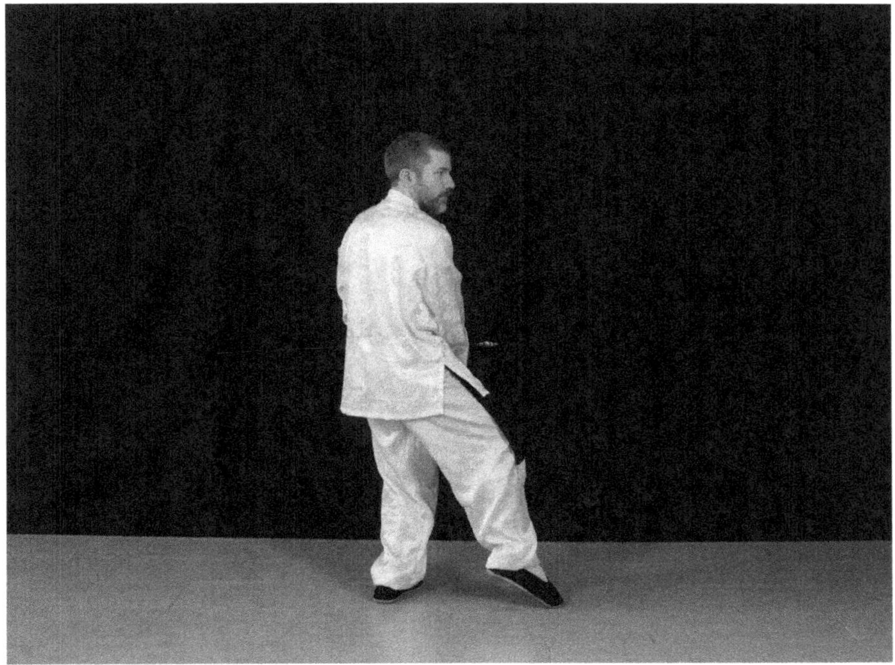

EAST. Bring the grip of the sword closer to your solar plexus, placing the index and middle fingers of the left hand on your right forearm. Open the step laterally with your right leg, placing the right foot slightly forward in terms of the left one. As you shift your body weight from the left leg, execute a horizontal cut, followed by the turn of the waist with the sword blade in the *pingmian* position. At the end of the technique, the tip of the sword is facing north. It is necessary to apply a small correction to the toes of the left foot, turning them slightly to the right during the turn of the waist, to avoid damaging the knee ligaments.

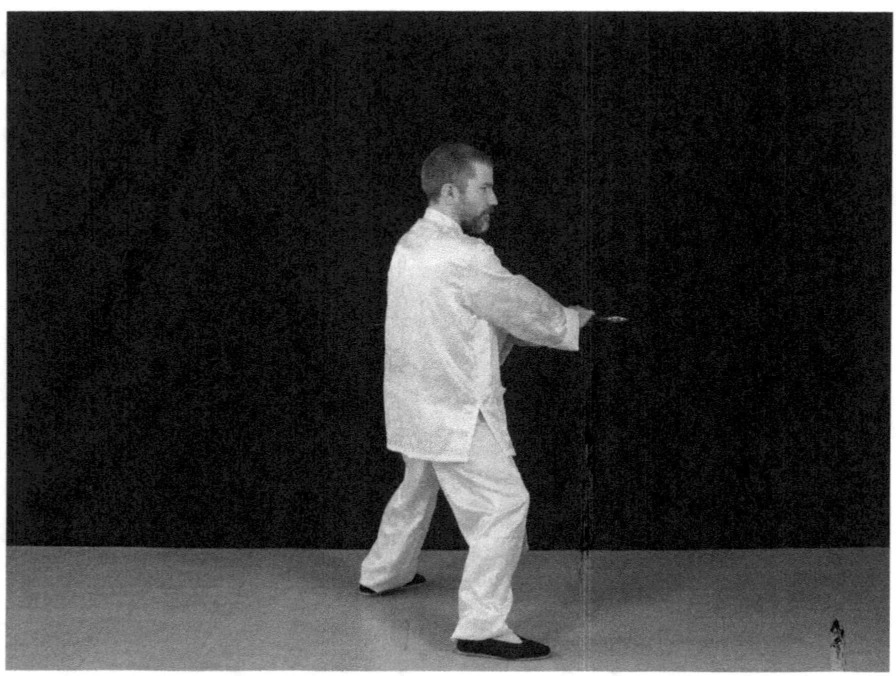

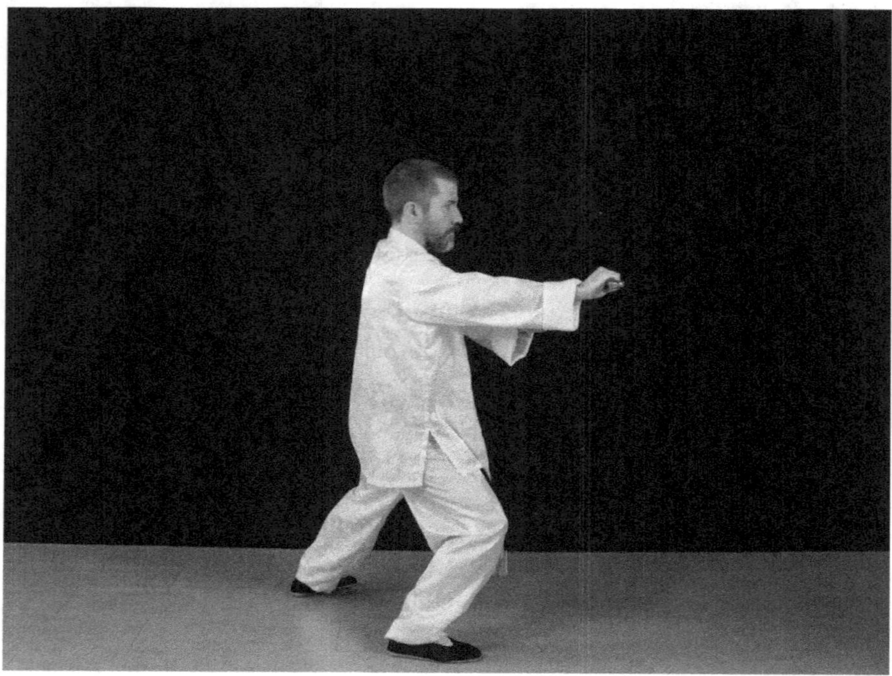

11
The wind blows the lotus leaves - 烏龍擺尾

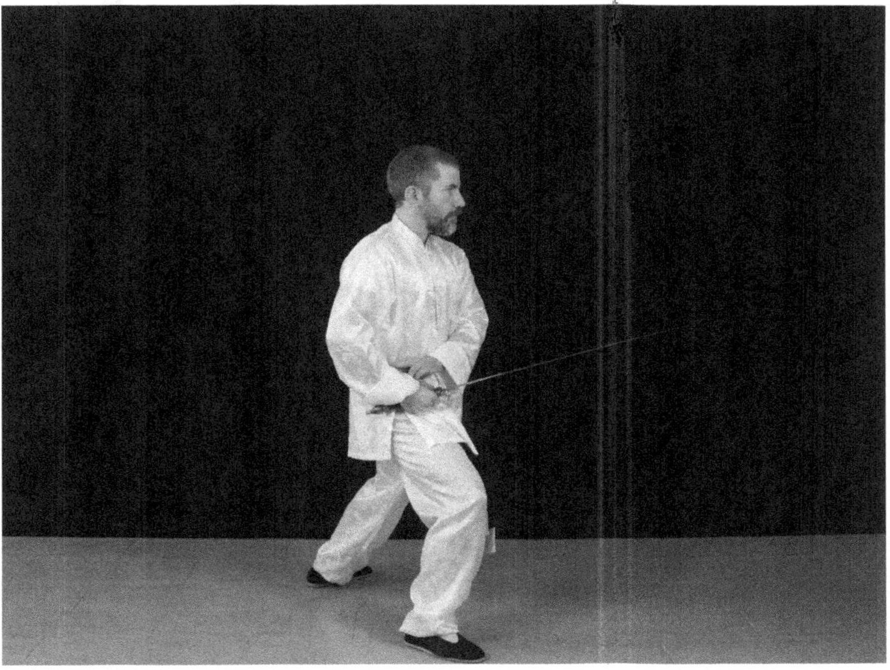

EAST. Bring the sword to your right hip, keeping the secret sword on your left forearm. Turn your right wrist clockwise at one hundred and eighty degrees. From this preparatory position, execute a straight thrust to the east. The left hand must be placed on the left flank above the head.

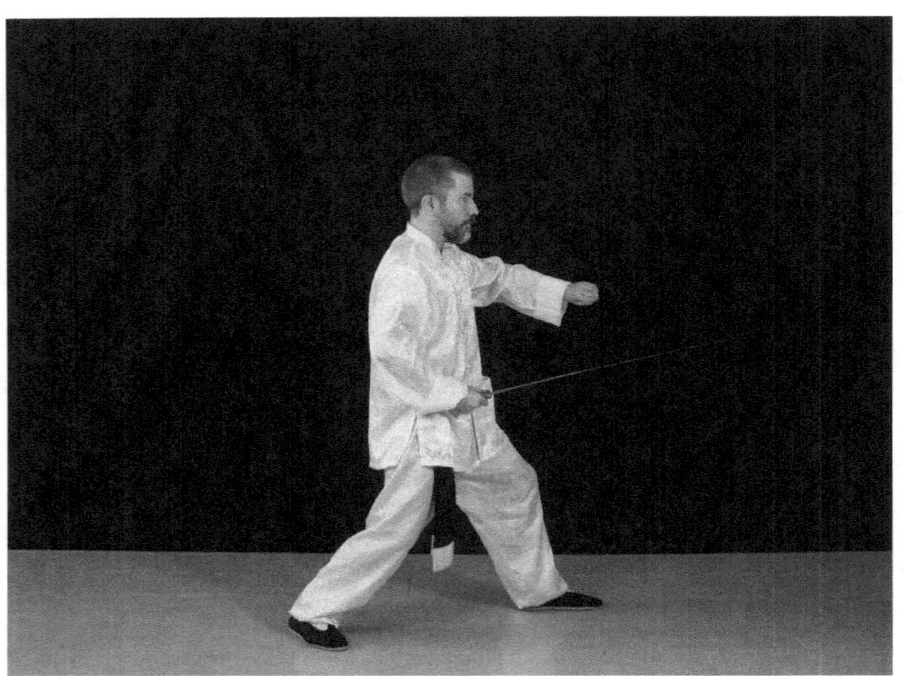

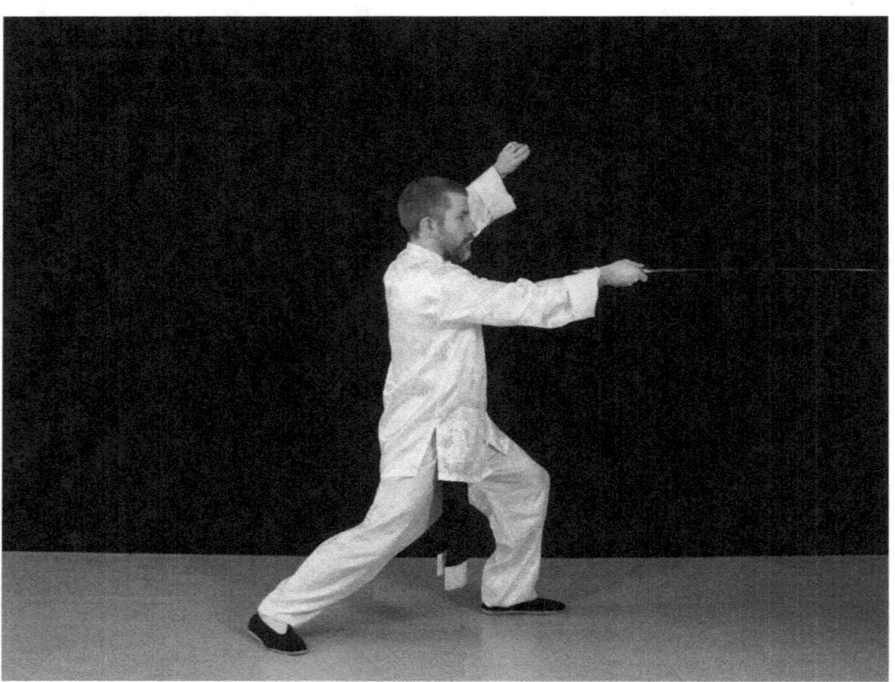

12
The lion shakes its head - 夜叉探海

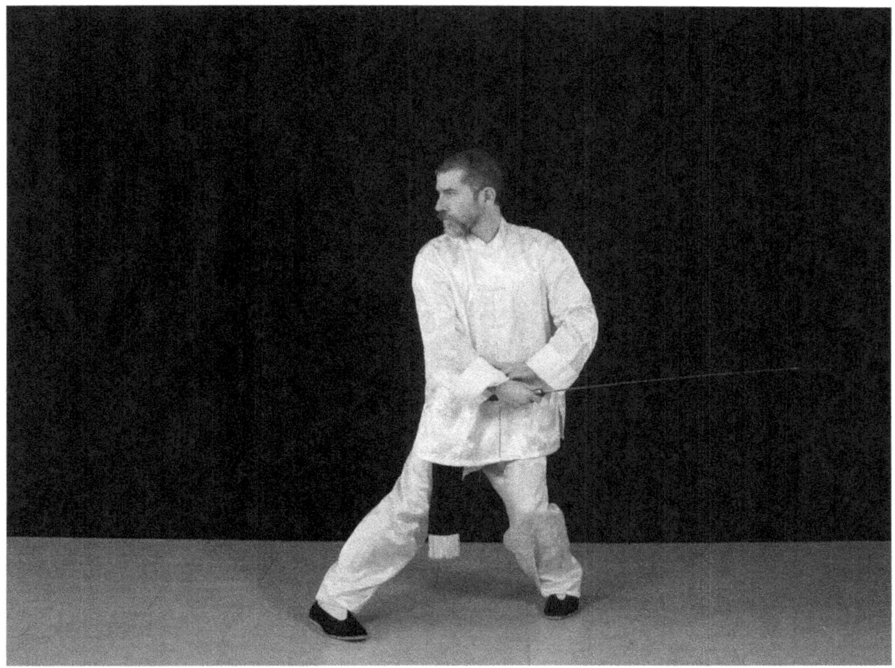

WEST. Transfer most of your body weight to the right leg, bringing the sword to the starting position of the previous technique. Then, turn one hundred and eighty degrees to the right pivoting on the left heel. Shift the weight to your left leg. In continuation, raise your right leg, directing your right foot toes towards the ground. At the same time as the right leg is lifted, turn your right wrist to the left, so that your palm ends up face down.

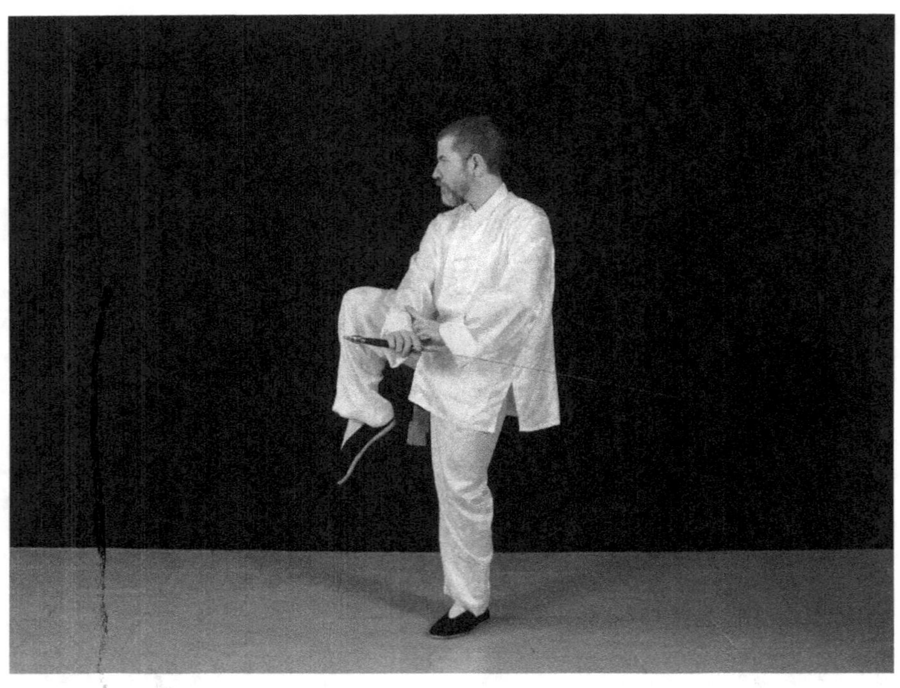

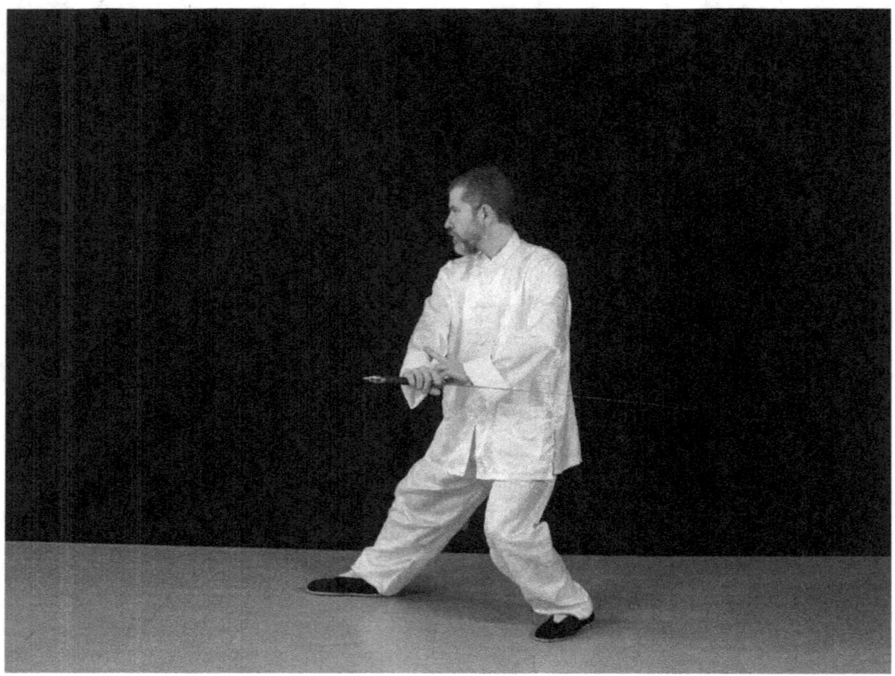

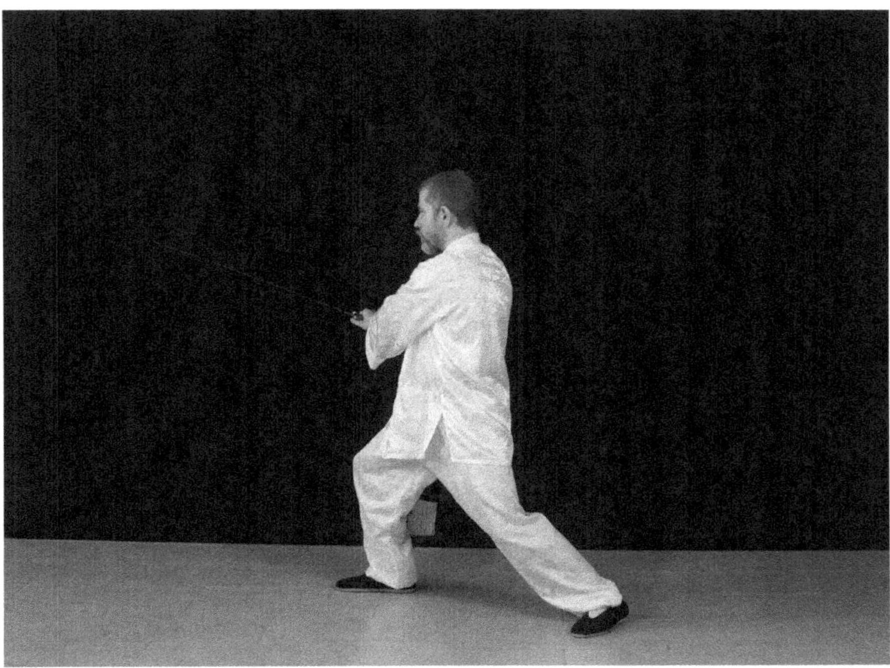

Step into the right bow stance. The sword describes a curved trajectory, performing a cut forward accompanied by the turn of the waist. At the end of its trajectory, the tip of the blade points to the west. The index and middle fingers of your left hand rest on the right forearm.

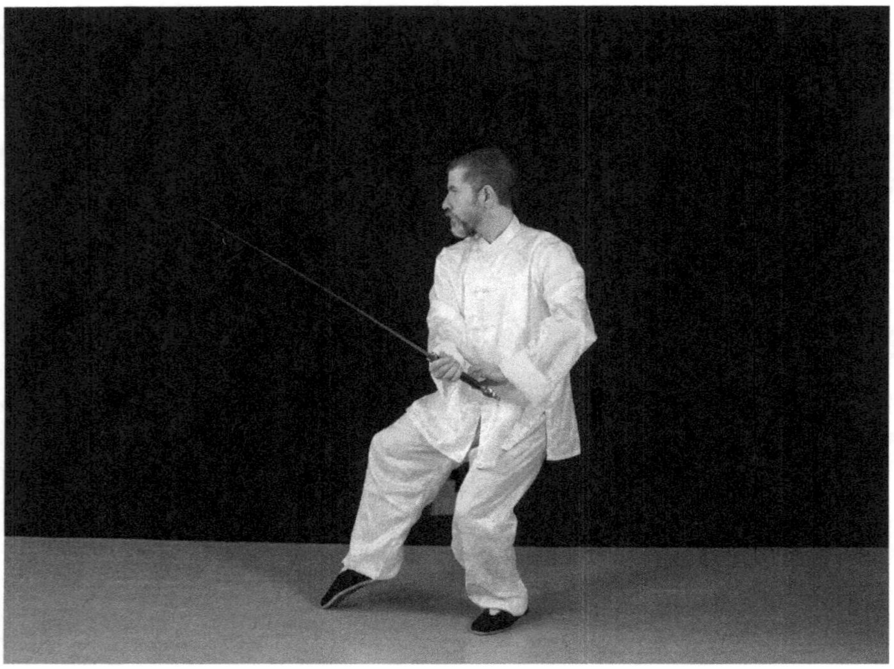

Step back with the right foot, into the middle step of the preceding bow stance. Turn your wrist one hundred and eighty degrees to the right so that the sides of the sword blade are inverted, still in the pingmian position. While the turn of the waist and the shift of the weight to the left leg are taking place, the sword performs a cut in reverse, analogous to the previous one. At the end of the cut, the tip of the sword points to the west.

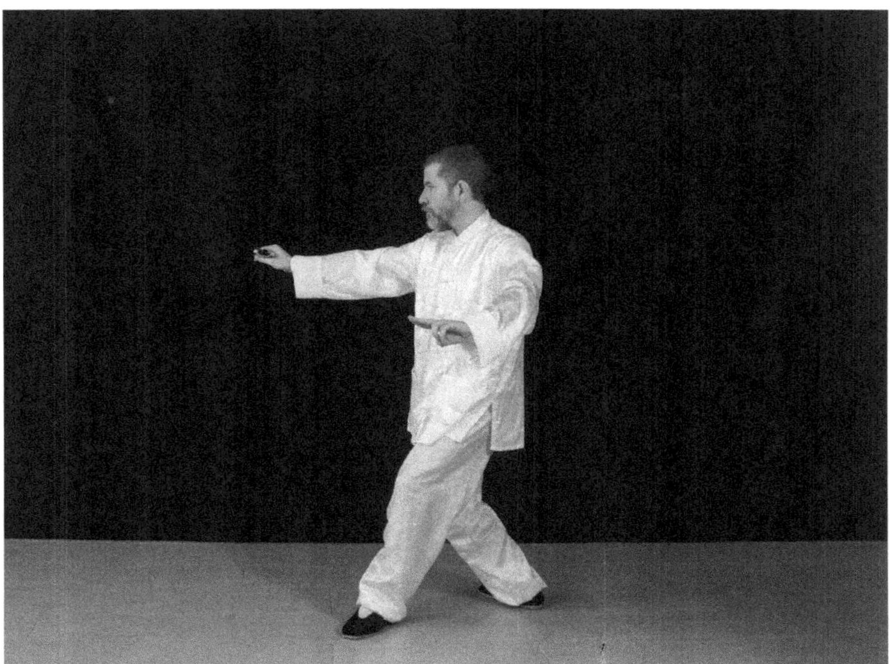

Take a step backwards with your right foot to form a middle step symmetrical to the previous one. From the centre of the torso, separate your hands to describe an outward arc. The tips of the secret sword and the Gim should converge at the same point in front of your face, forming a triangle. At the end of the technique, the hands are situated at a height no superior to that of the solar plexus and not inferior to that of the hip. The steps of this sequence of cuts remind us of those performed in the technique *Repulse monkey*, even though it would be imprecise to say that they are identical.

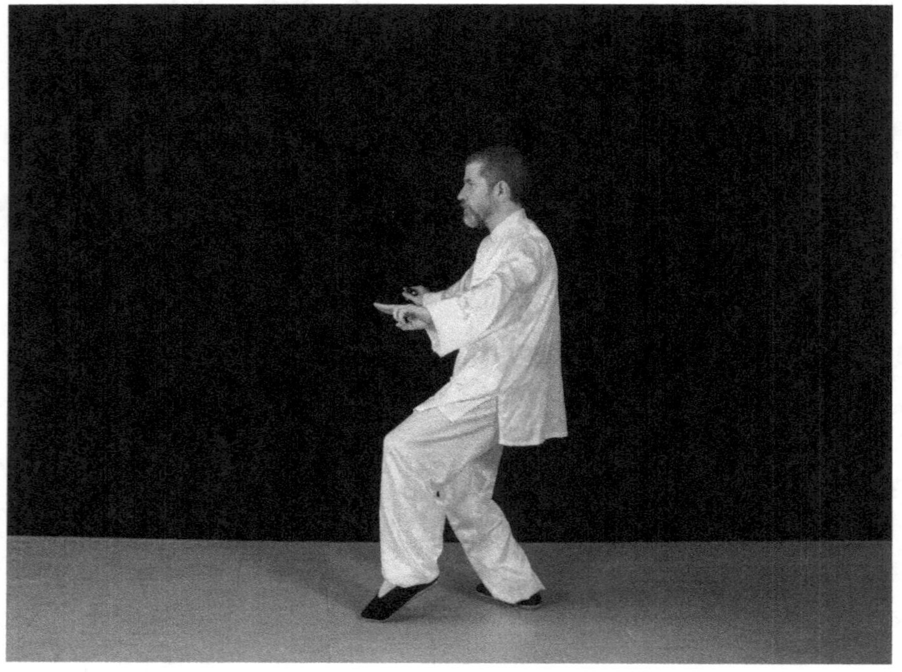

13
The tiger raises its head - 虎抱頭

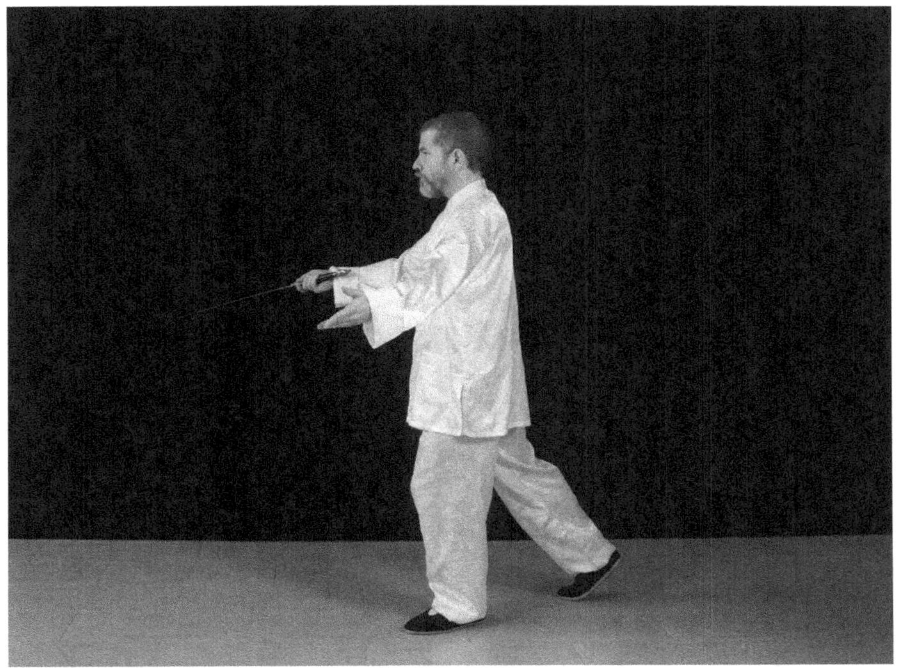

WEST. After turning both wrists one hundred and eighty degrees, both hands are in the centre of the body, in front of your solar plexus. The right hand rests on the left palm. The sword is kept in *pingmian* pointing to the west. Raise your right leg, maintaining the toes facing down.

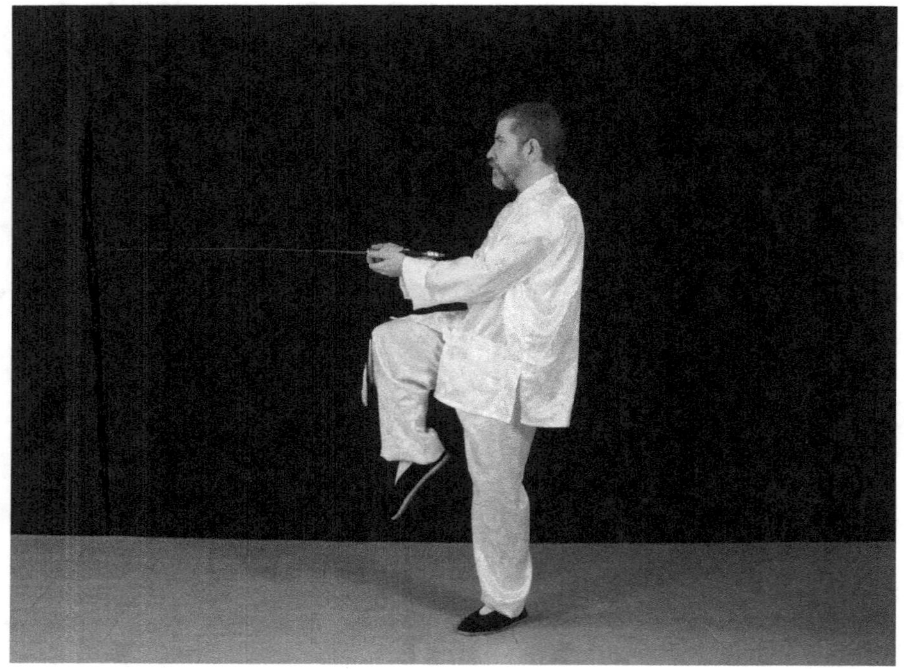

14
The wild horse jumps over the creek - 野馬跳澗

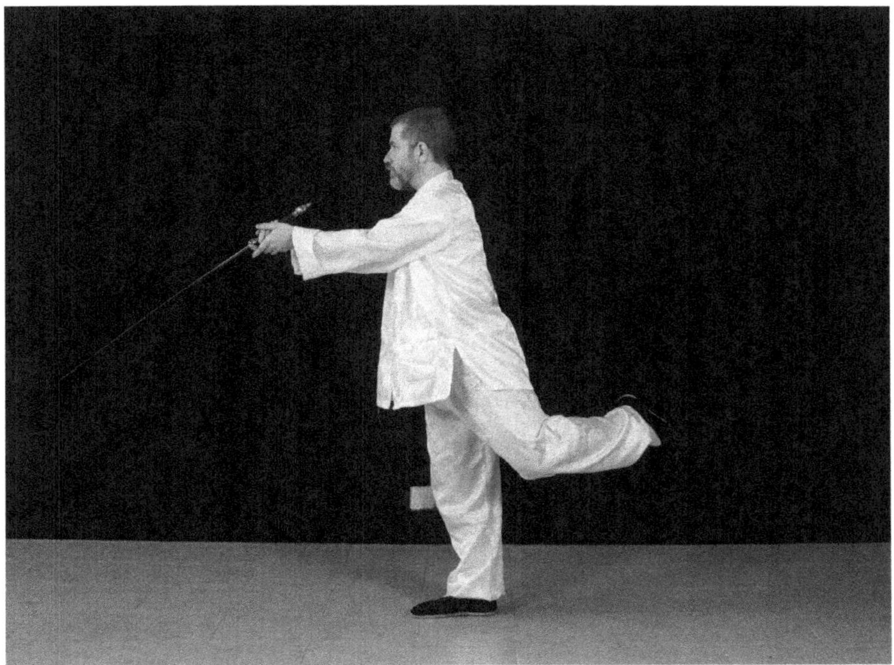

WEST. Rest the right foot on the ground, slightly extending your elbows and letting the point of the sword softly bend downwards. From this position, jump to the west gaining momentum from the right leg. The left foot establishes contact with the ground first, the toes ending up facing southwest. Step forward into the right bow stance. Then, execute a thrust to the west keeping the sword in *pingmian*. The left hand is placed above the head on the left flank.

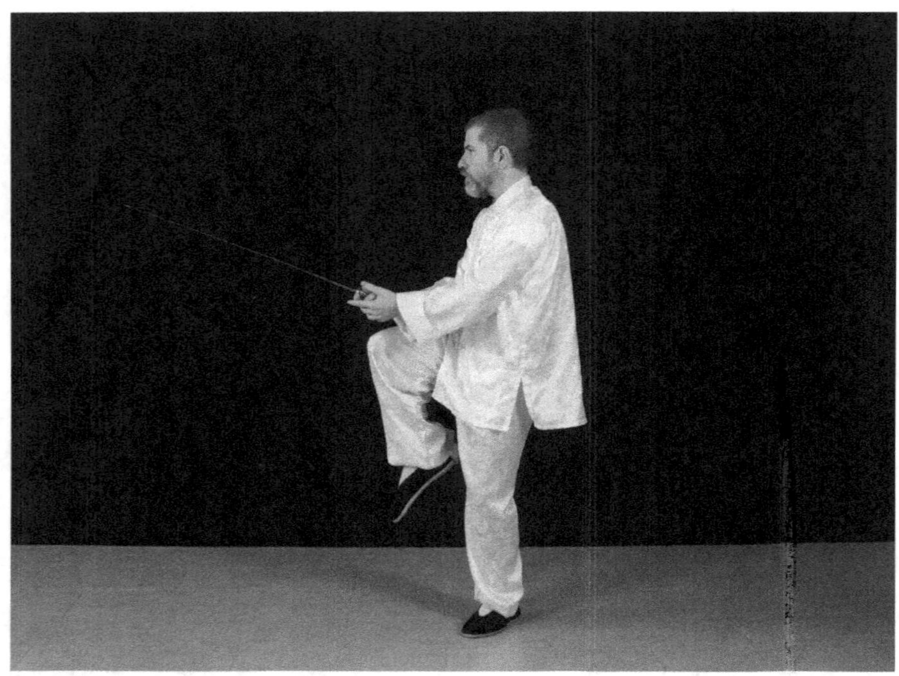

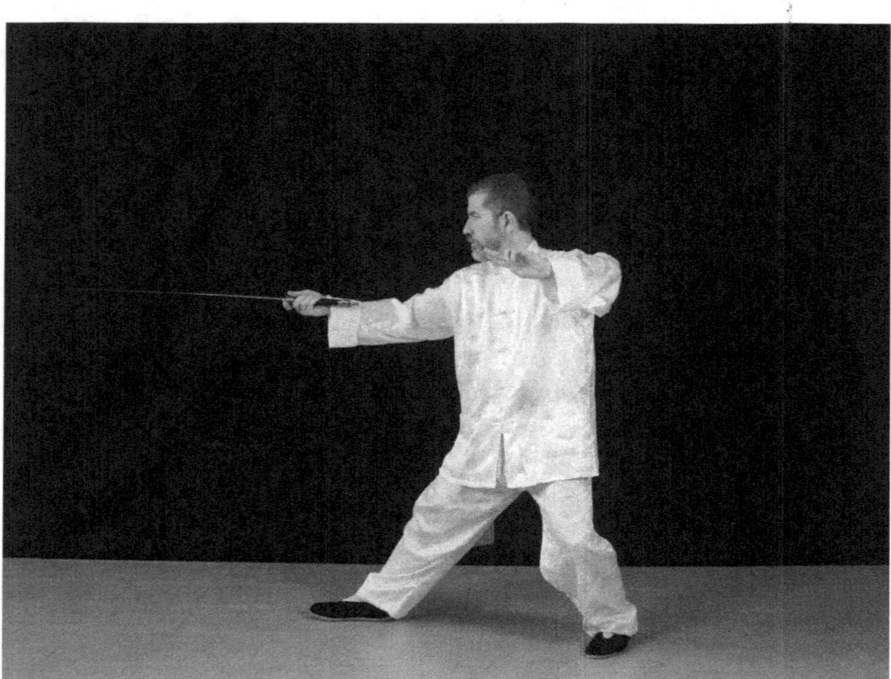

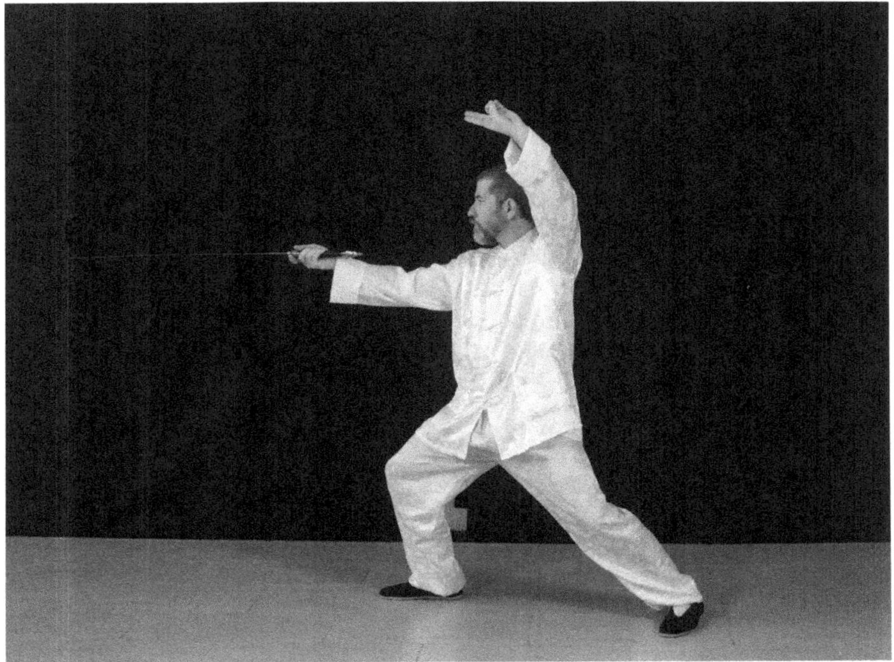

15
Little star of dipper - 小魁星

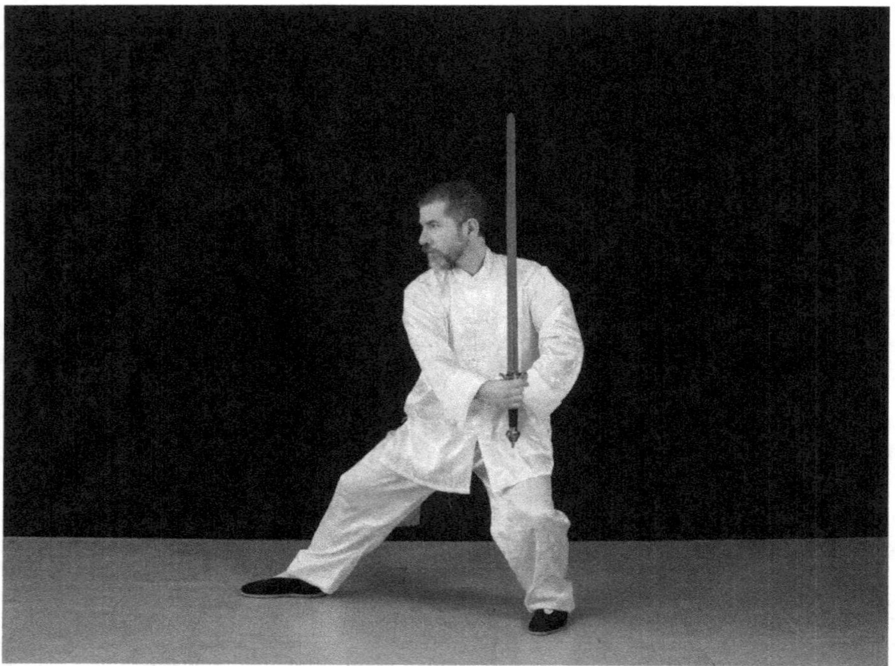

WEST. Transfer most of the body weight to your left leg. During the weight shift, the sword draws a descending arc counter-clockwise. Turn your waist to the left. As the hilt approaches the height of your left shoulder, the index and middle fingers of your left hand should be placed on your left forearm. During the execution of the movement, turn your right wrist to the left to place the sword in the *zhimian* position.

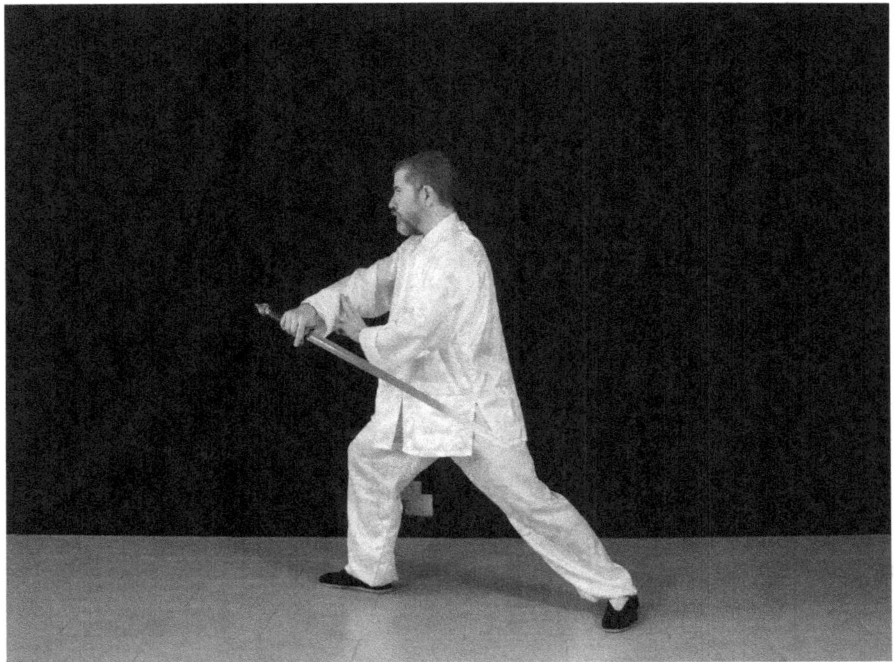

Then, open the right foot toes forty-five degrees and advance with the left foot into the middle step of the bow stance. The body weight rests on your right leg. During the advancement, the cut varies its route and undertakes an ascending trajectory in front of the torso. At the end of the movement, the tip of the sword points downwards at a forty-five-degree angle. The left hand has not been separated from the forearm.

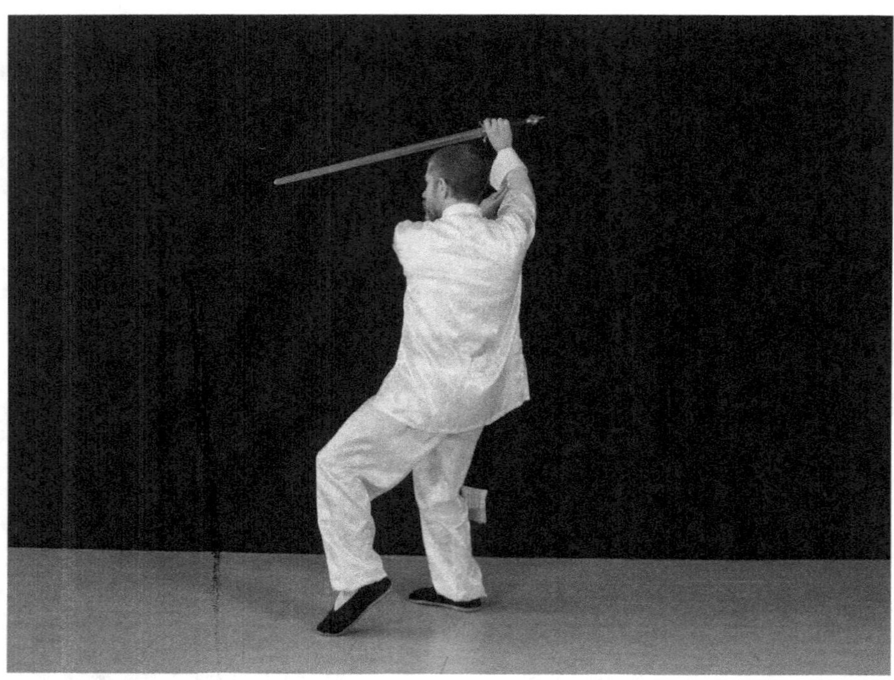

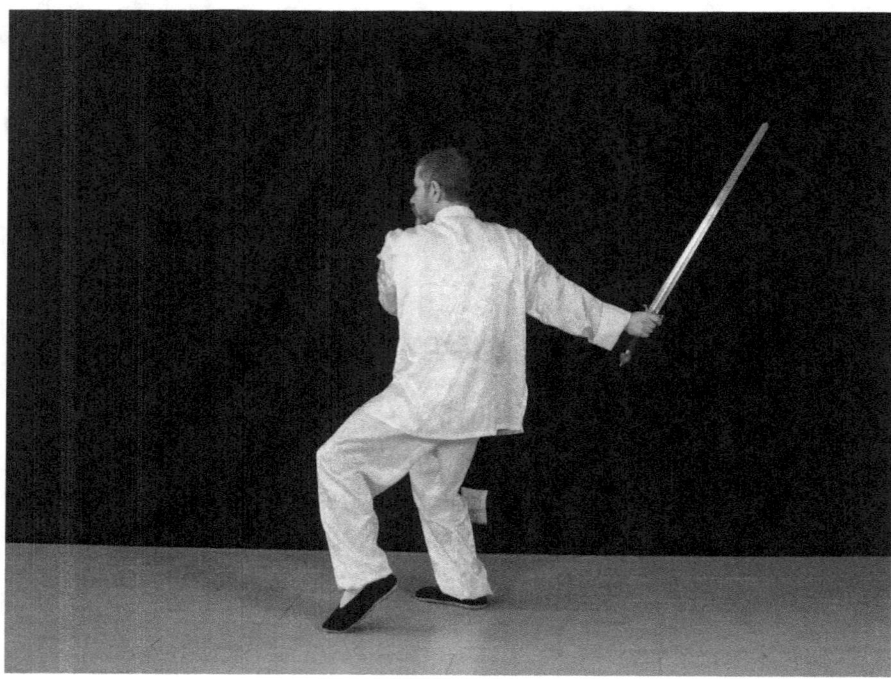

16

Fishing the moon out from the bottom of the sea - 海底撈月

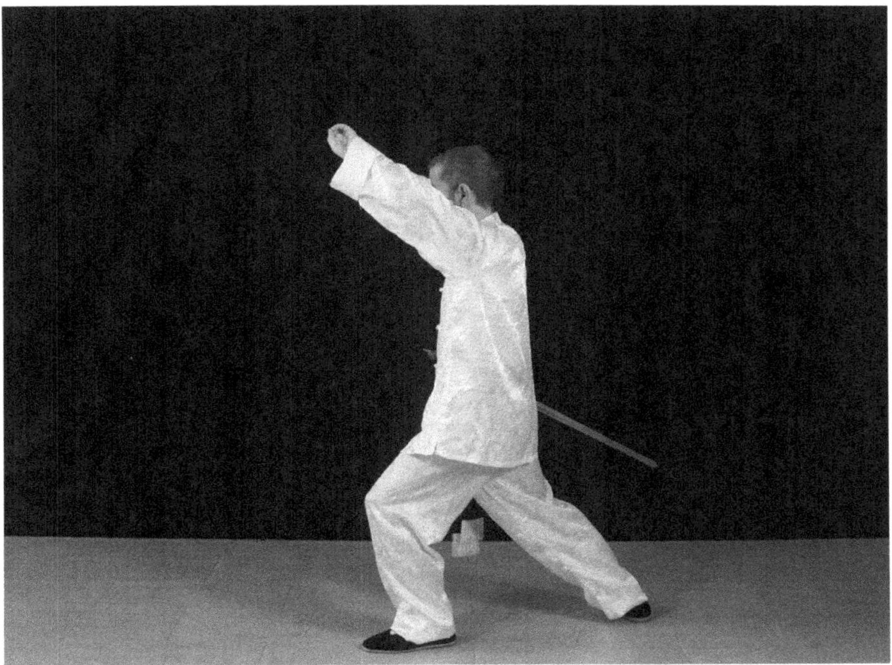

WEST. In this technique, the practitioner performs a wide cut accompanied by the turn of the waist maintaining the blade of the Gim in the *zhimian* position. From the final position of the previous technique, step forward crossing with the left foot to get into the right bow stance. During the step forward, the sword draws an ascending arc from behind, finalising its trajectory parallelly to the ground. The secret sword is placed above the head, on the left flank.

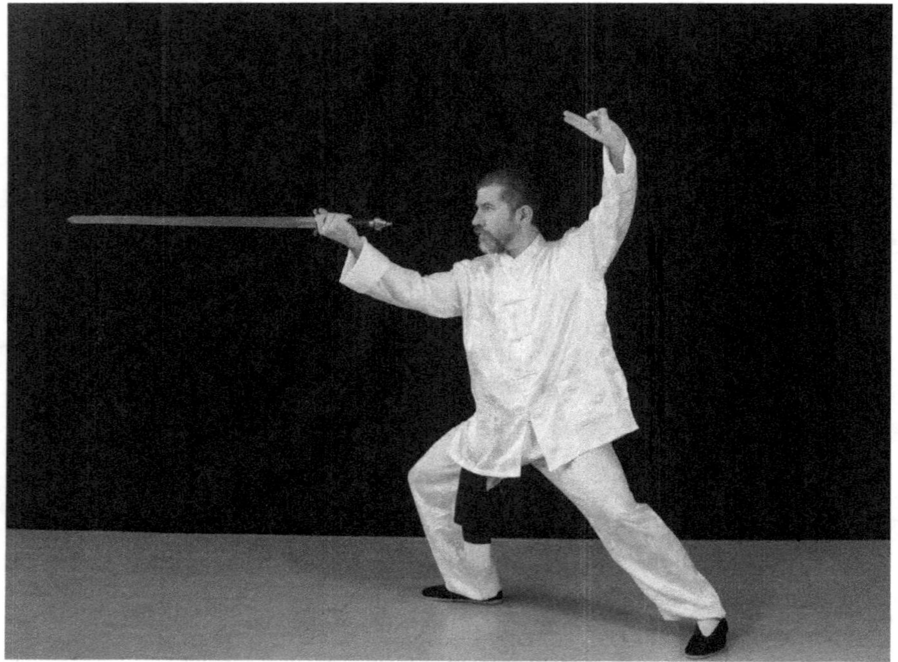

17
The rhinoceros gazes at the moon - 犀牛望月

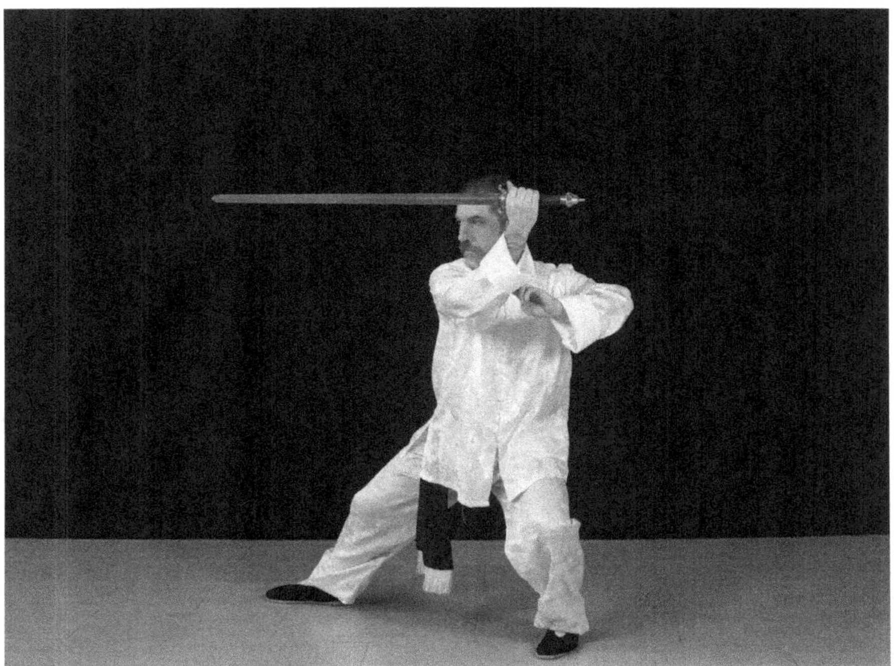

WEST. Shift the body weight to your left leg, moving the sword from the right side to the left without modifying its angle. The waist turns to the south. At the end of the movement, the sword is at the height of the left temple. The index and middle fingers of the left hand are rested on the interior part of the right forearm.

Shooting the wild goose - 射雁势

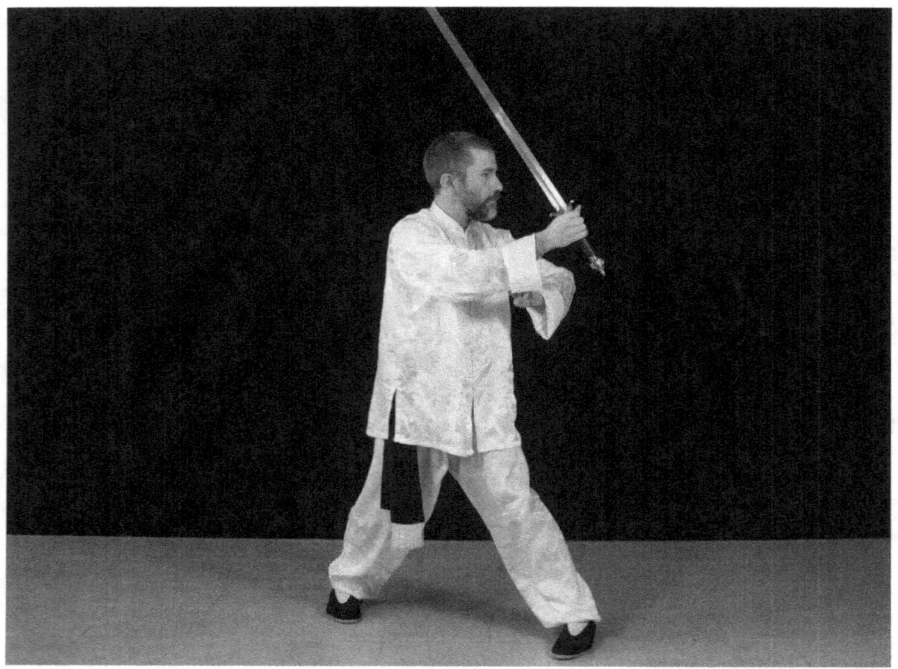

EAST. Pivot on the right heel to get into the middle step of the bow stance. Most of the body weight rests on the right leg. In the middle step, the sword performs a vertical turn downwards, the tip stopping at a position slightly tilted to the ground.

Then, the secret sword is separated from the forearm and points east. The waist turns to the right. The sword comes down until it is placed on the right hip, maintaining the *zhimian* position.

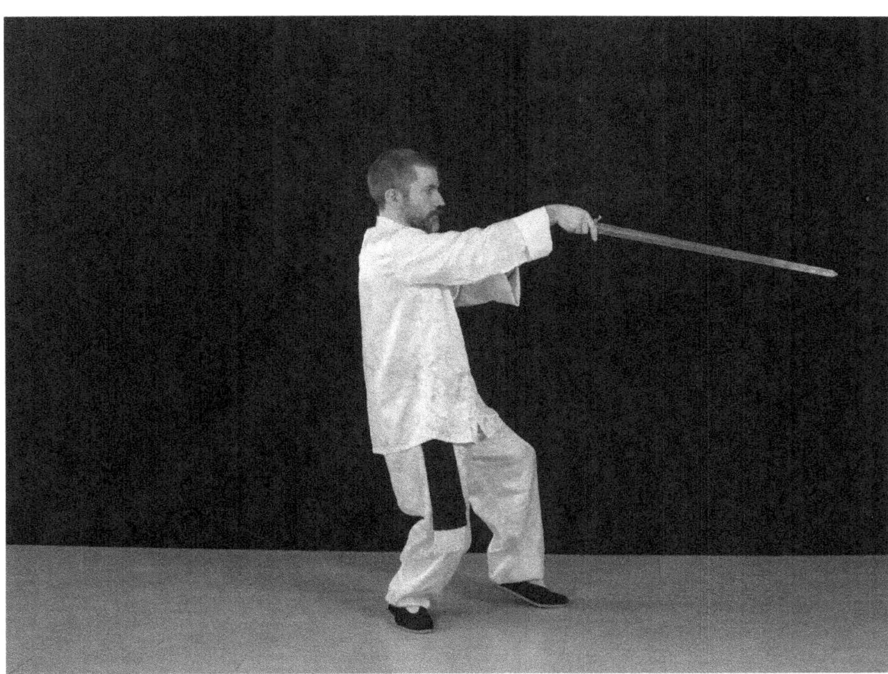

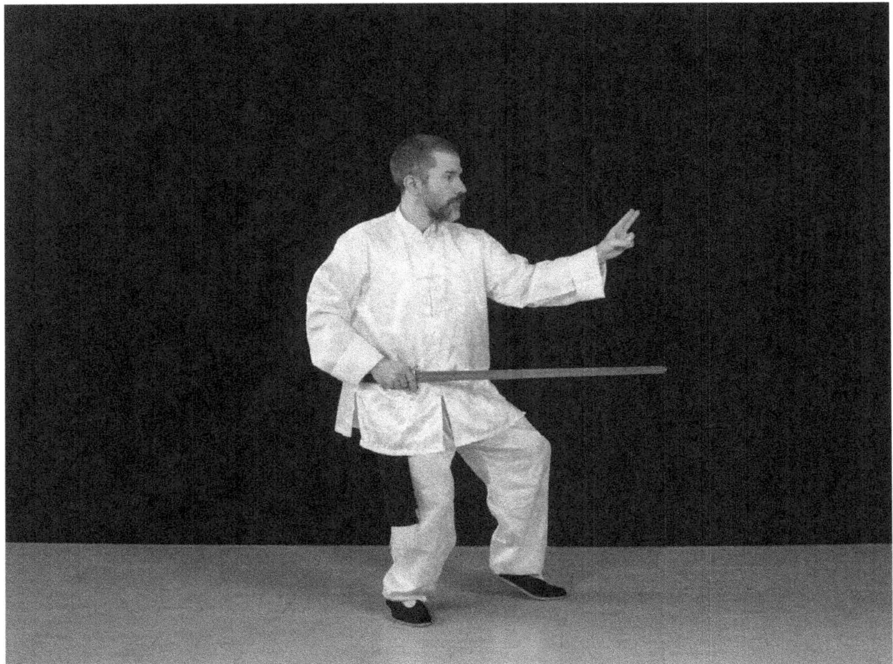

18
The white ape offers the fruit - 白色猴子提供果子

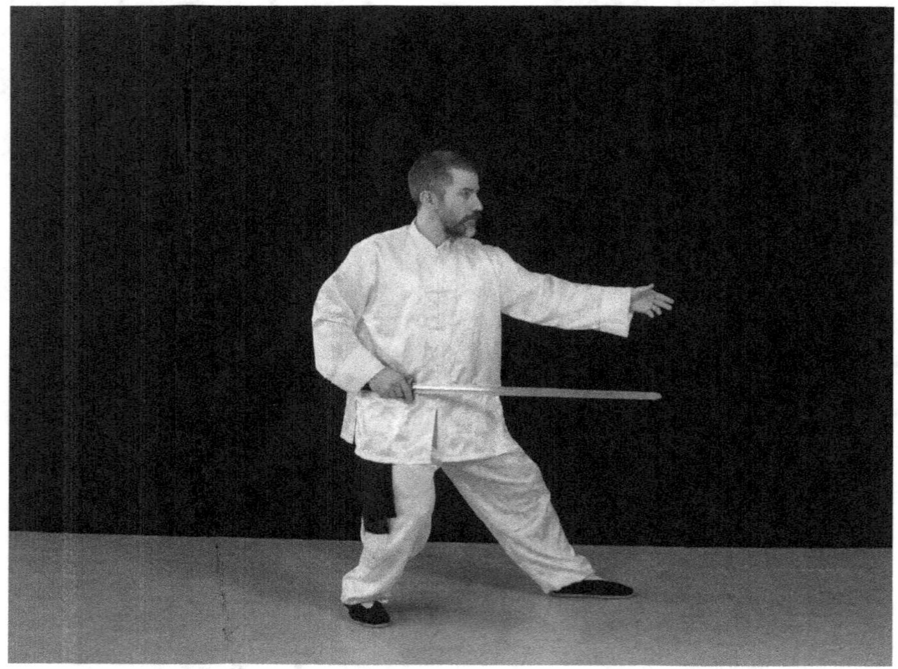

EAST. Advance east with your left foot, and reposition the right one so that both feet are joined together. Straighten your knees. Turn your right wrist ninety degrees to the right to place the sword blade in the *pingmian* position. Execute a horizontal thrust to the east, maintaining the Gim at a height slightly inferior to that of the shoulders. The right hand rests on the open palm of the left one.

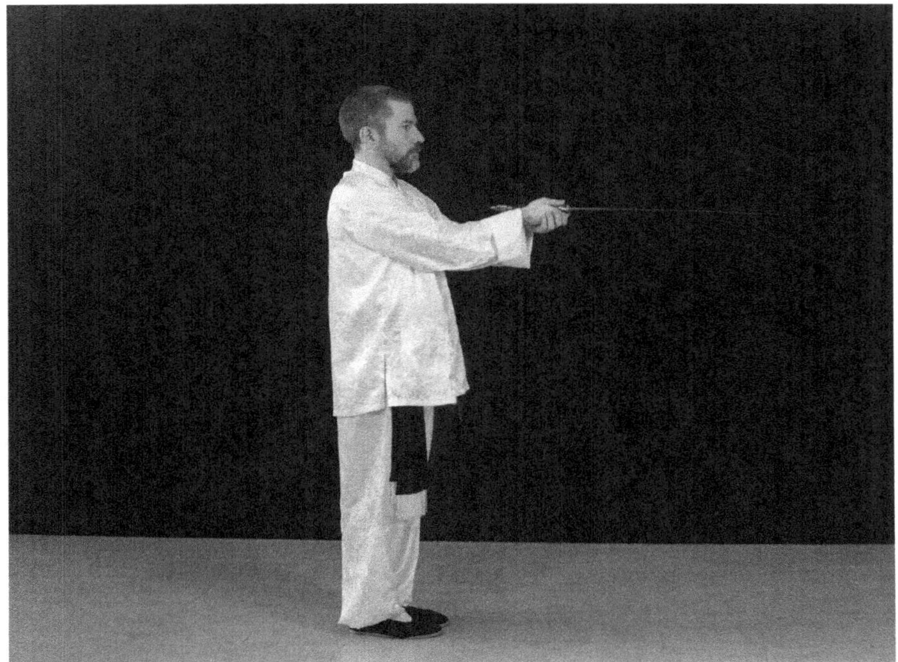

19
Dusting in the wind, left - 迎風揮塵左

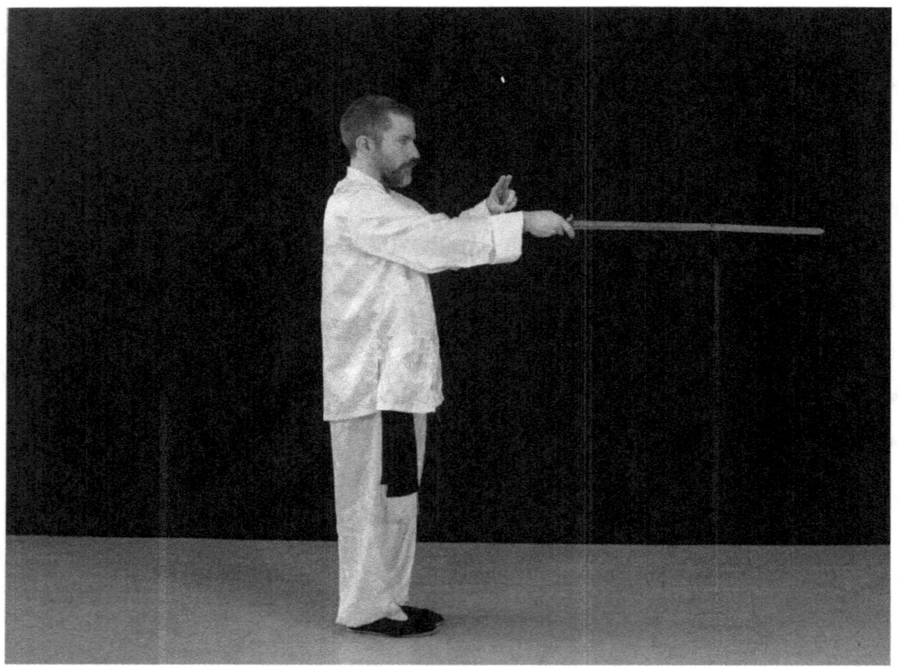

EAST. Bend your knees. Turn your right wrist ninety degrees to the left to place the sword in *zhimian*. At the same time, open your right foot toes forty-five degrees and turn the waist to the right at the same angle. Then, place most of the body weight on your right leg and advance with the left leg into the bow stance. During the movement, the sword describes a wide arc from behind, starting the cut on the right flank, and ending it on the left one. The waist turns accompanying the entire movement. The left hand ends up above the head on the left flank. This technique bears resemblance to *The fair lady works the shuttle*.

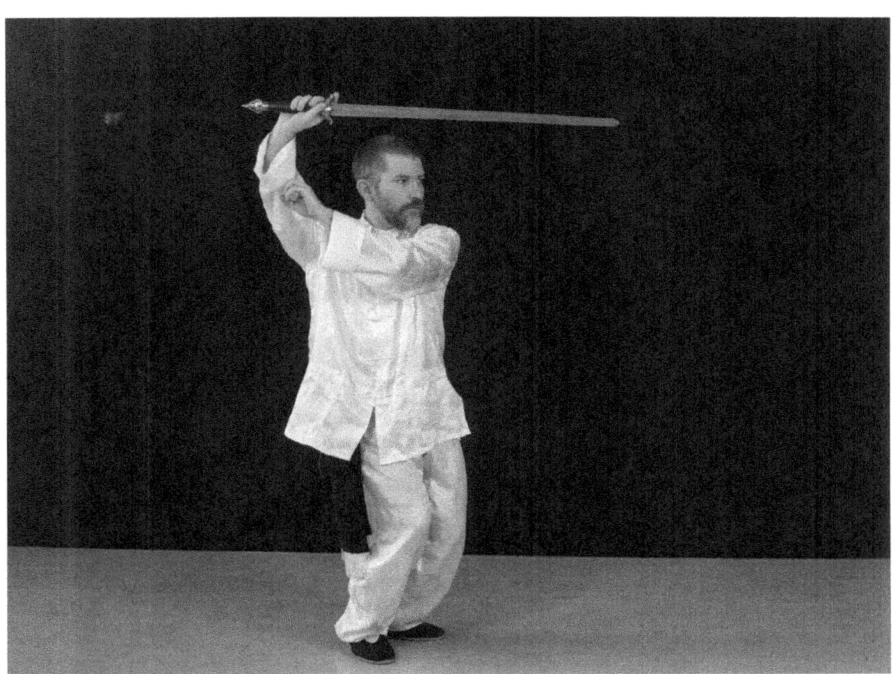

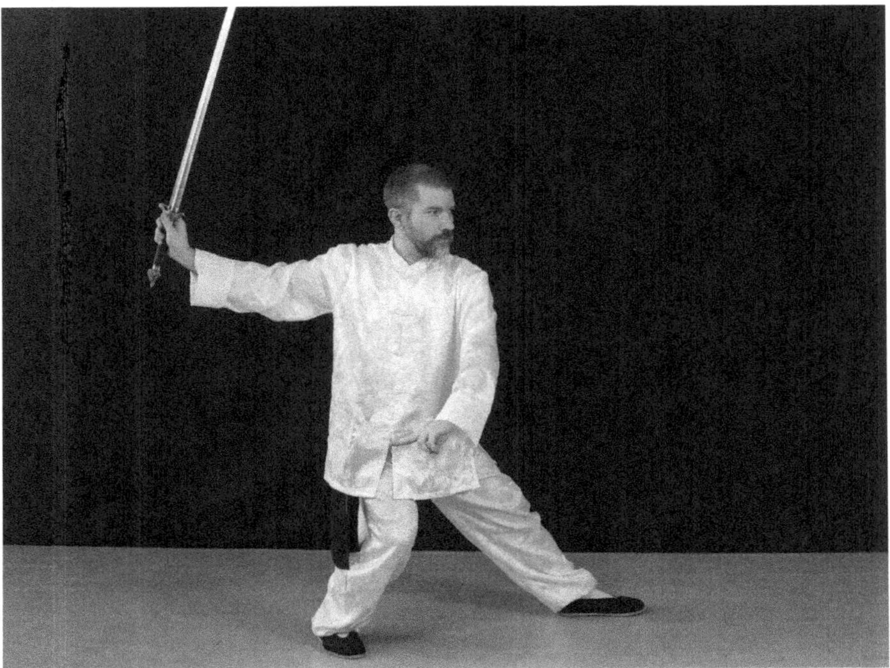

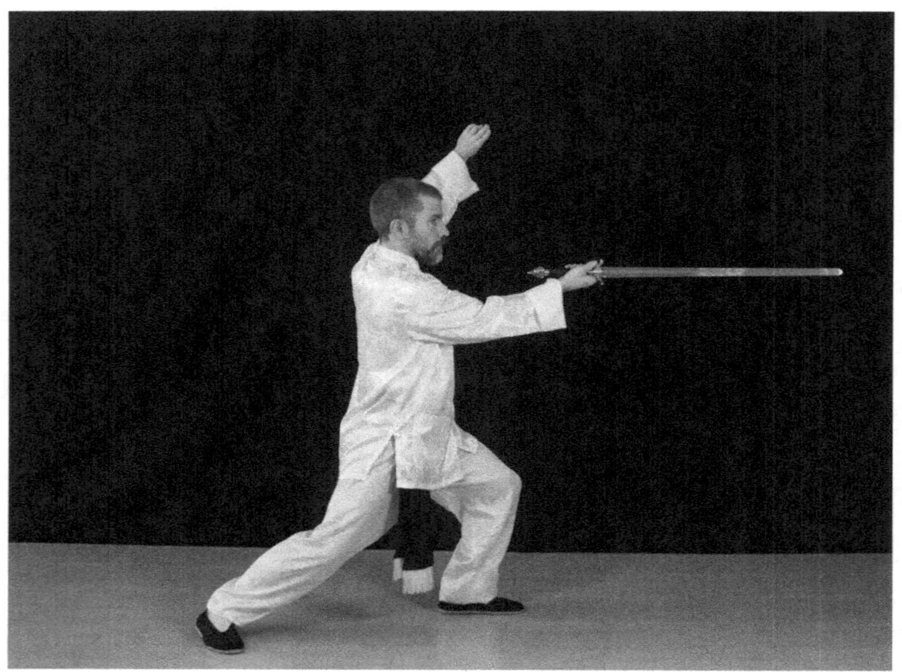

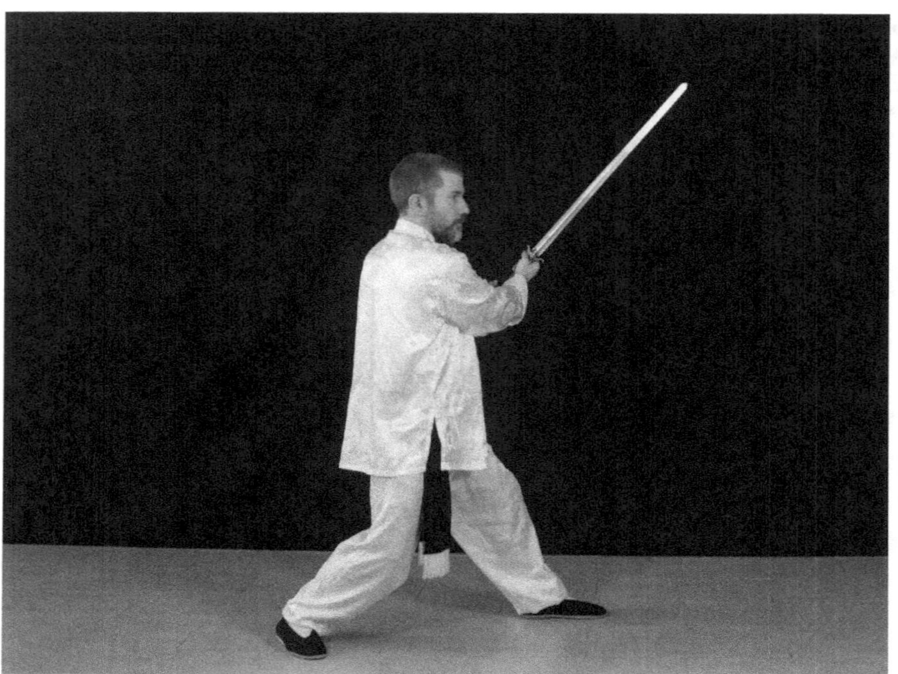

20
Dusting in the wind, right - 迎風揮塵右

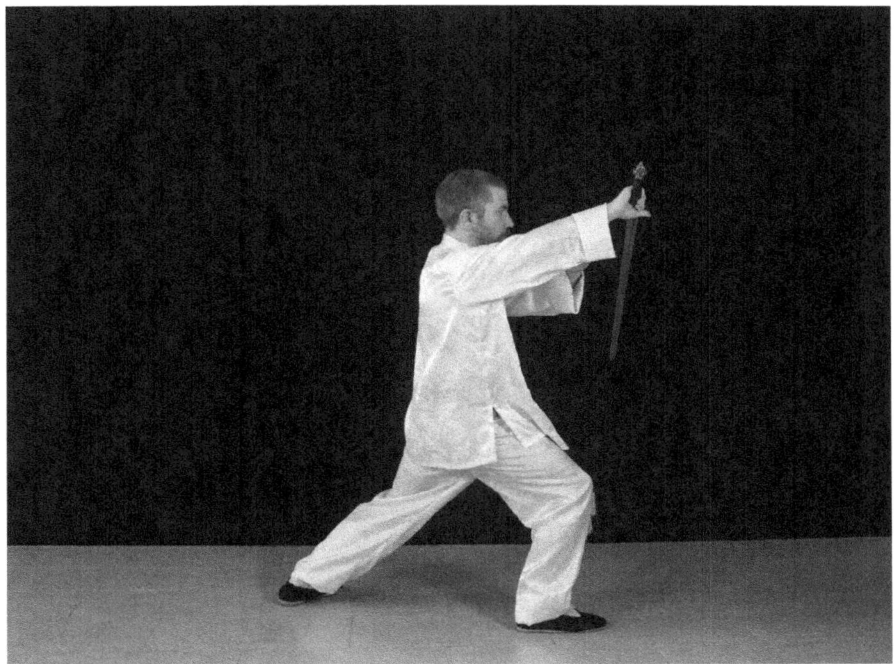

EAST. Step forward into the right bow stance. The index and middle fingers of the left hand are placed on the right forearm. The sword performs an ascending frontal cut, accompanied by the rotation of the waist, at a forty-five-degree angle.

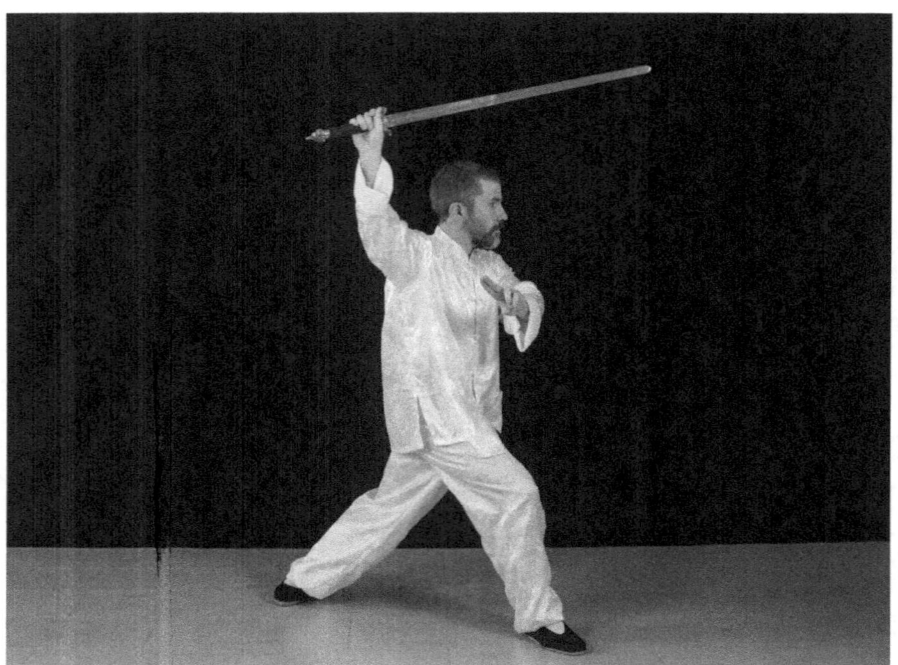

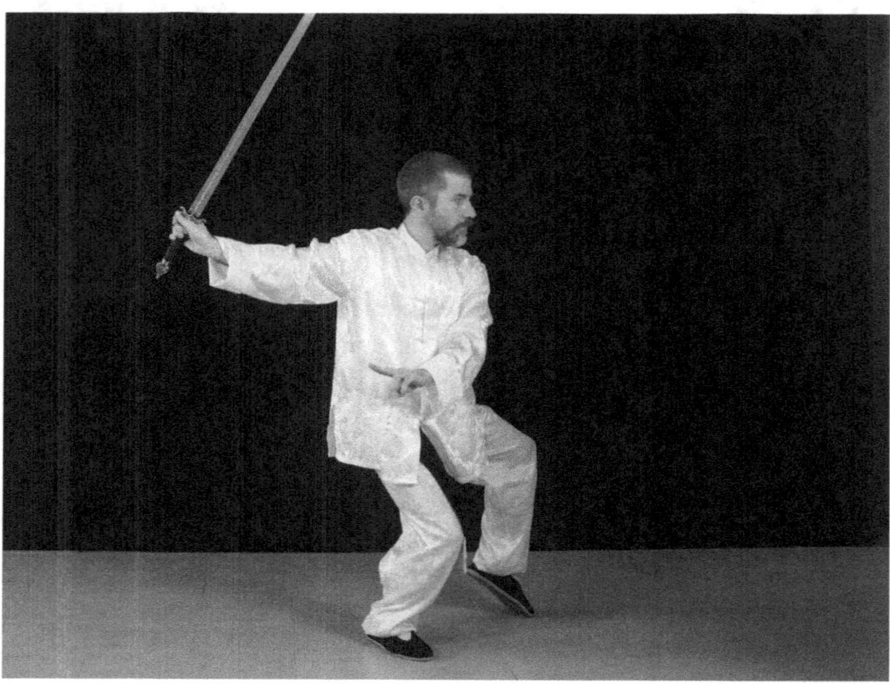

<h1 style="text-align:center">21</h1>

Dusting in the wind, left - 迎風撣塵左

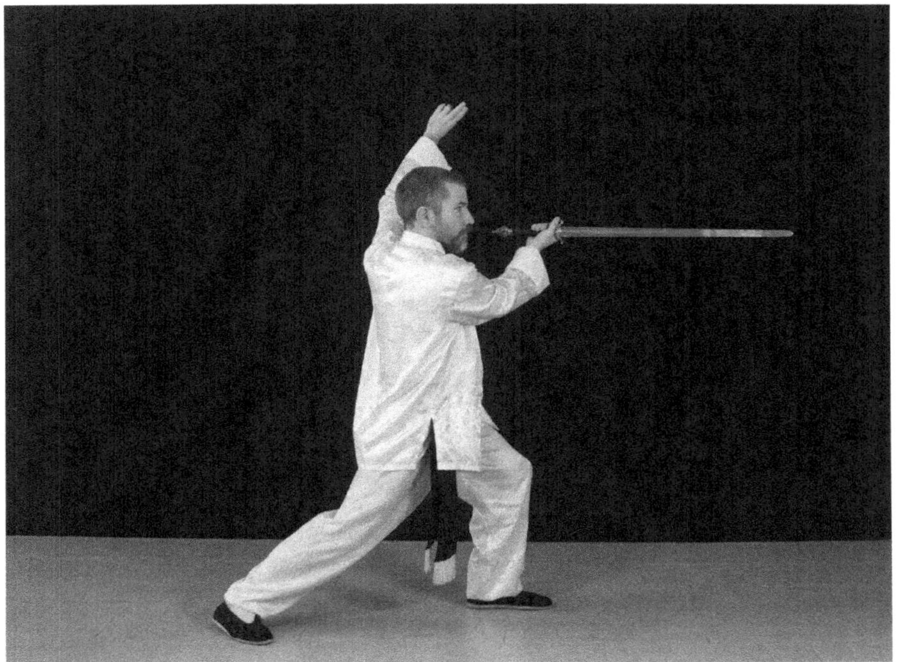

EAST. From the end of the previous cut, step forward into the left bow stance. Following the natural trajectory of the sword, repeat the cut of technique number nineteen, which opens this sequence of three movements.

22
Push the boat with the current - 順水推舟

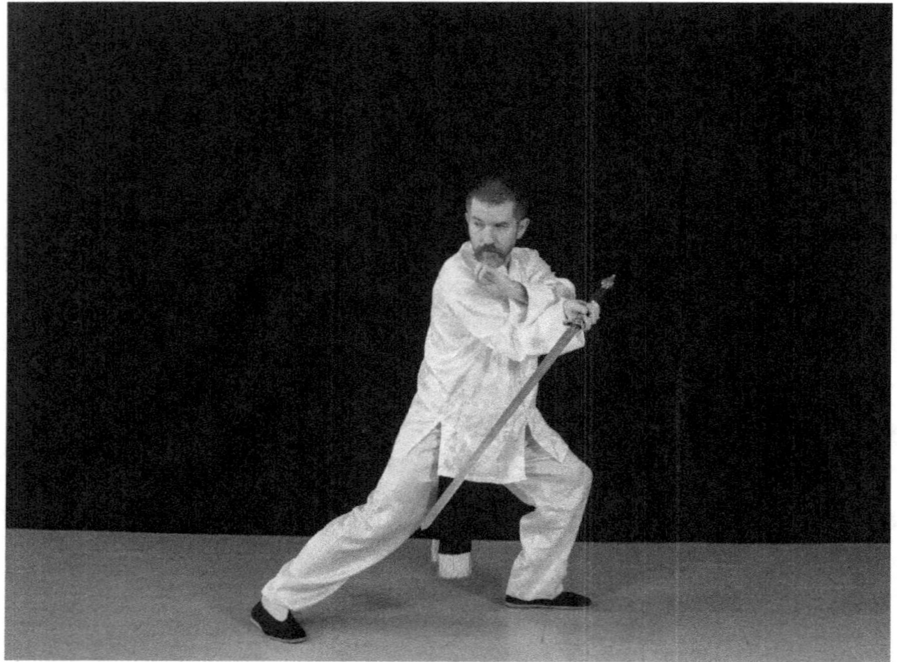

EAST. Direct the gaze to the west, bringing the secret sword to the right shoulder. The right hand holds the sword at the same angle as at the end of the previous technique, relaxing the wrist to allow for the next movement.

Next, advance to the east crossing your right leg in front of the left one in the way of quai ma. Execute a thrust to the west, maintaining the sword at the height of the shoulder in the *zhimian* position. The left hand ends up at the same height, with the fingers pointing to the east. The palms of both hands face south.

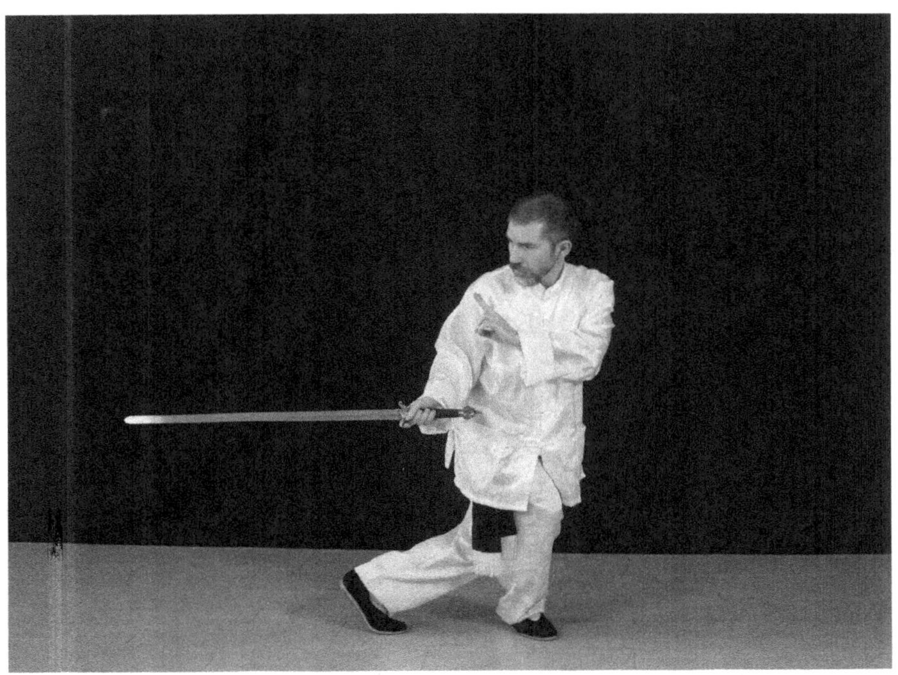

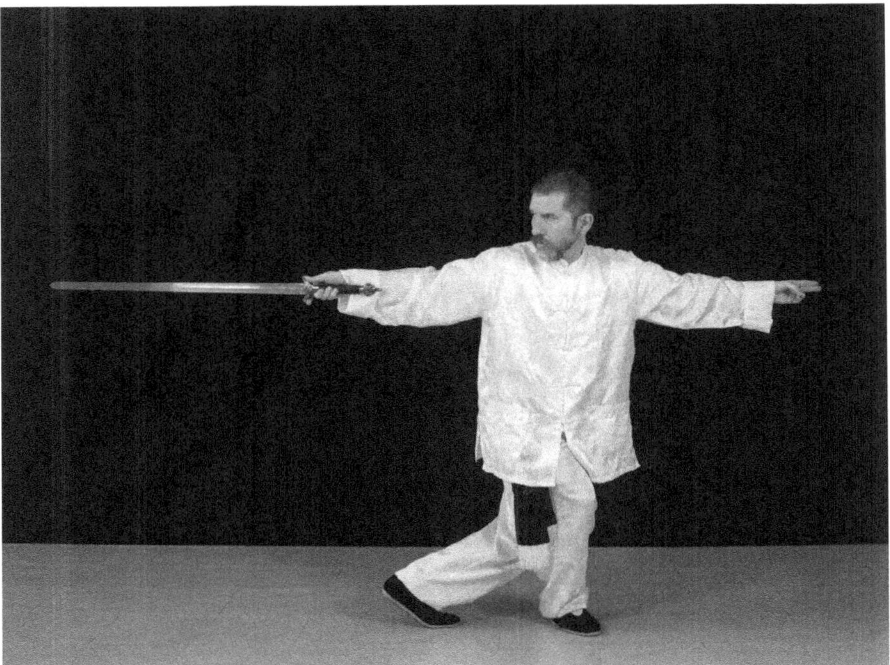

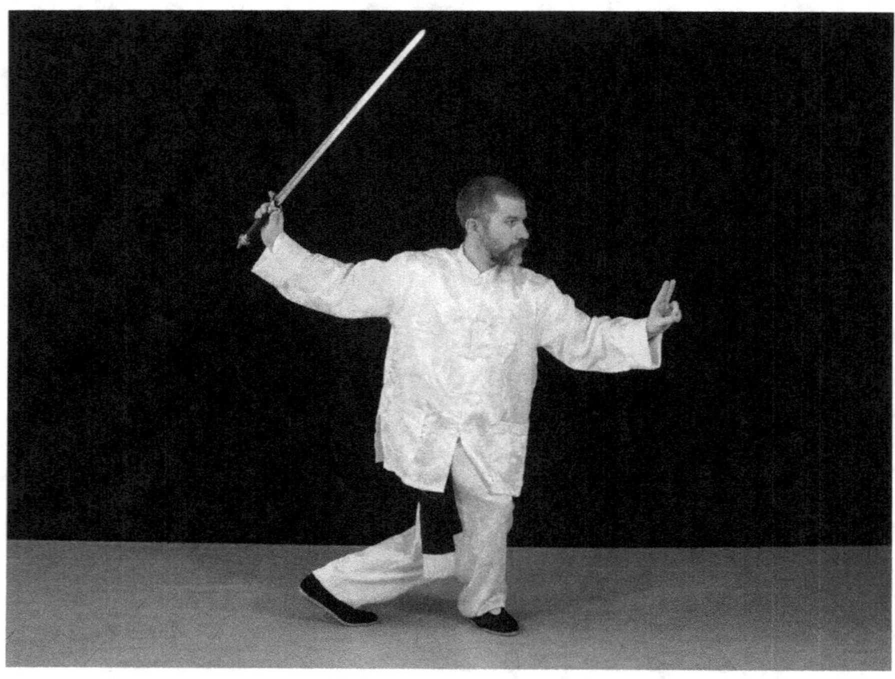

In the last part of the technique, advance to the east into the left bow stance, executing a descending thrust in the same direction, supporting it by rotating your waist. The point of the sword is facing down at a forty-five-degree angle. The index and middle fingers of your left hand rest on your right forearm.

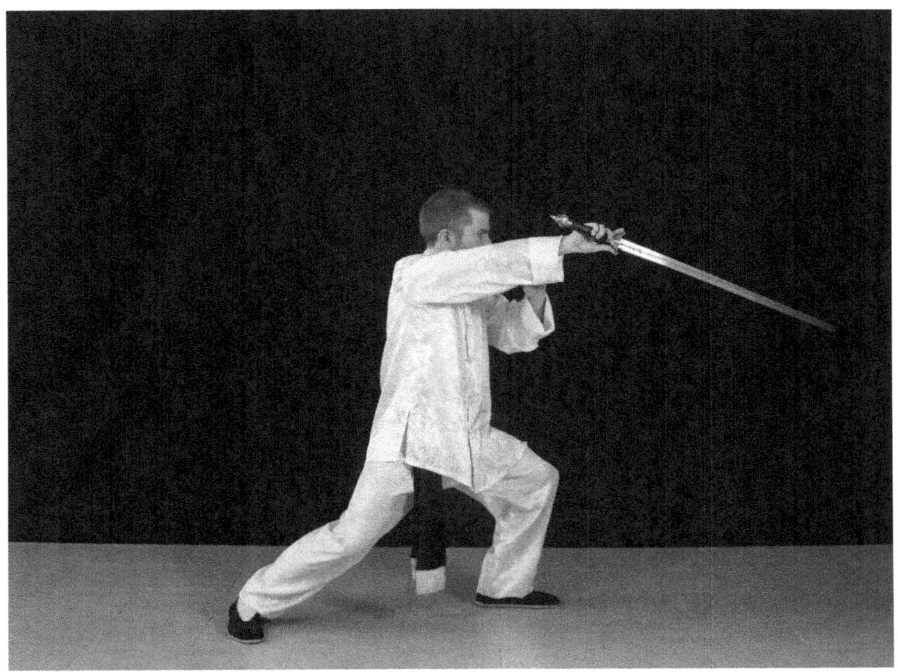

23
The comet chases the moon - 彗星飞行由月亮

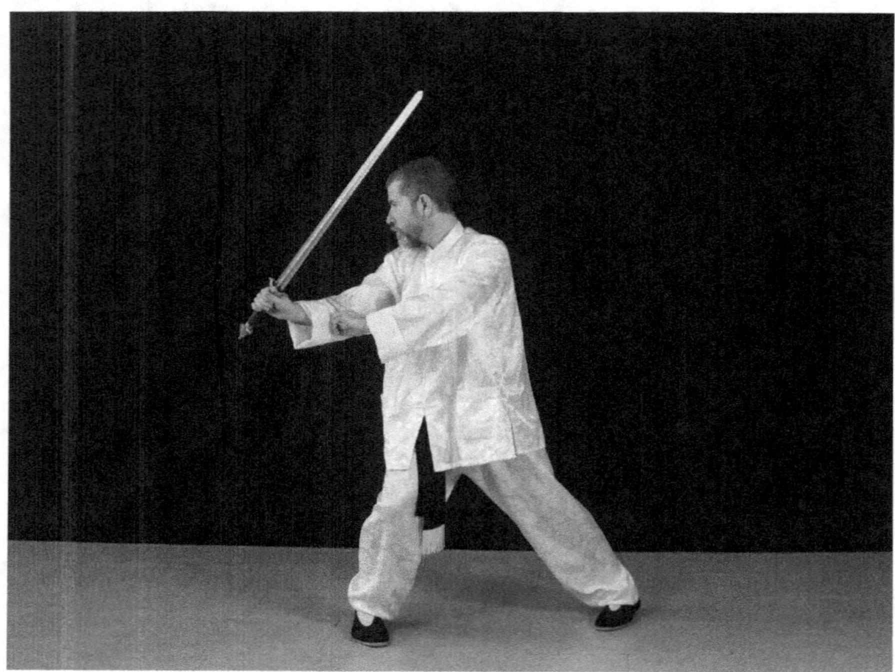

NORTHWEST. Shift the body weight to your right leg and pivot to the west on your left heel. The left foot toes are facing west. Step into the right bow stance. As the angle of the left foot toes reveals, it is a diagonal bow stance, in which the right foot toes point northwest. The sword executes a cut from above, the point of the blade ending up facing downwards at a forty-five-degree angle. To avoid losing control of the weapon, lower the hilt to the height of your solar plexus before performing the cutting part of the movement. Bring the secret sword above the head to the left flank.

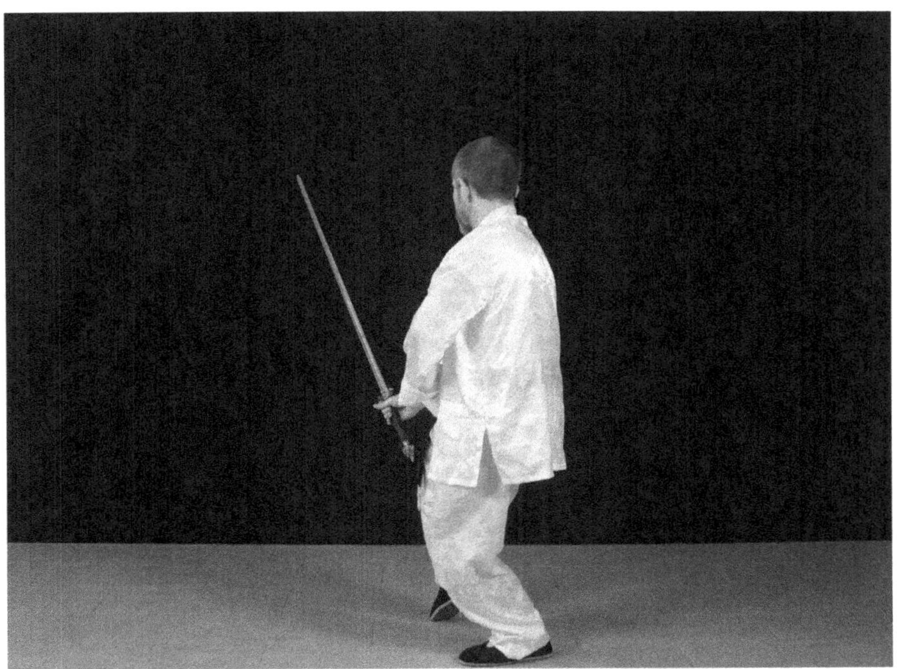

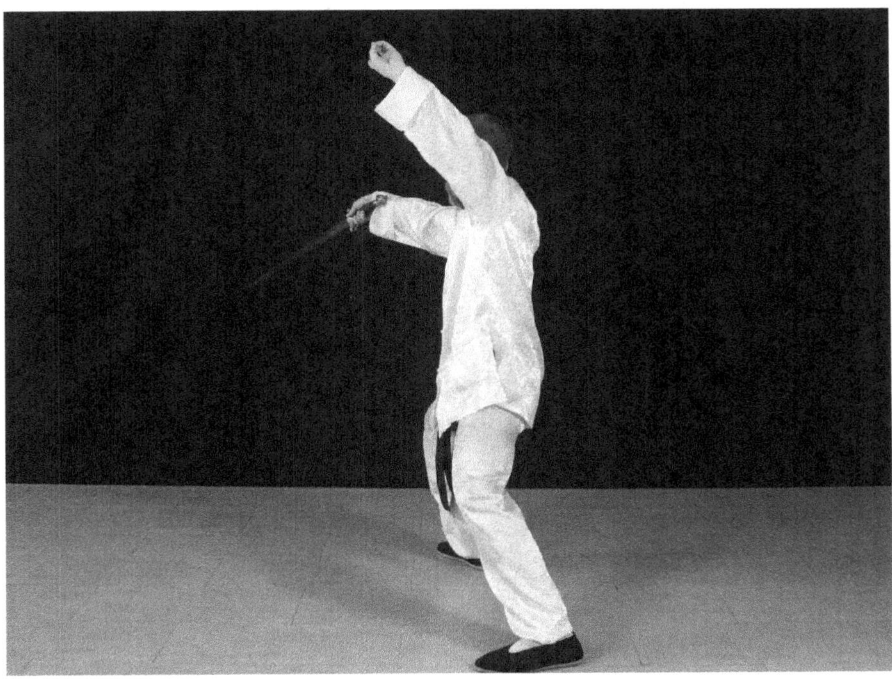

24
The celestial horse flies through the waterfall - 天马飞瀑

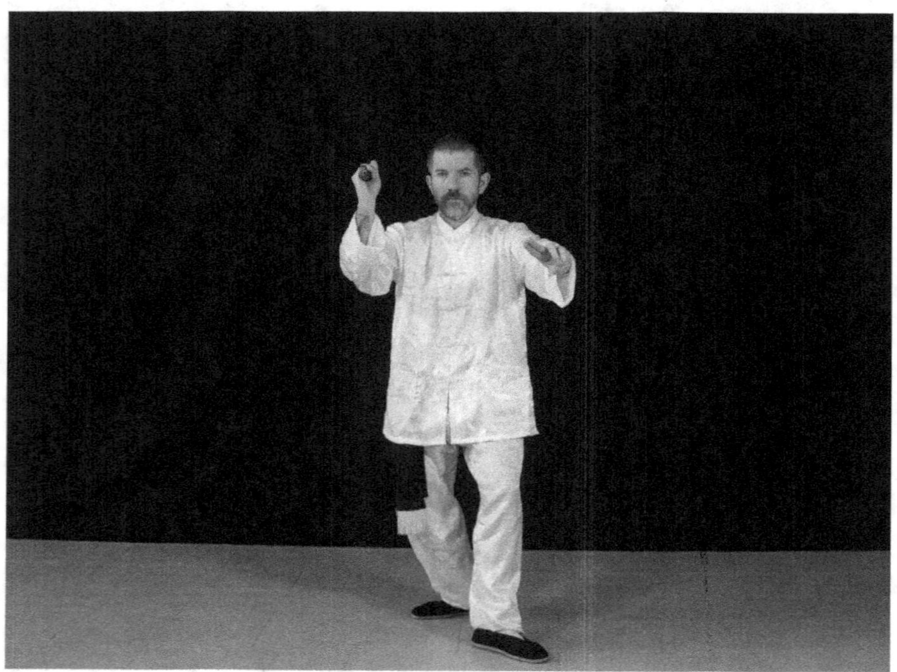

SOUTH. Advance with the left foot to the south, rotating on your left heel until the toes are facing southeast. Get into the middle step of the bow stance, placing most of the body weight on your left leg. The sword draws a descending arc over the right shoulder to perform a cut to the south. The point of the blade is facing down at a forty-five-degree angle. The right wrist turns ninety degrees to the left during the movement of the sword. The left hand makes a frontal circular clockwise movement, after which the index and middle fingers rest on the right forearm.

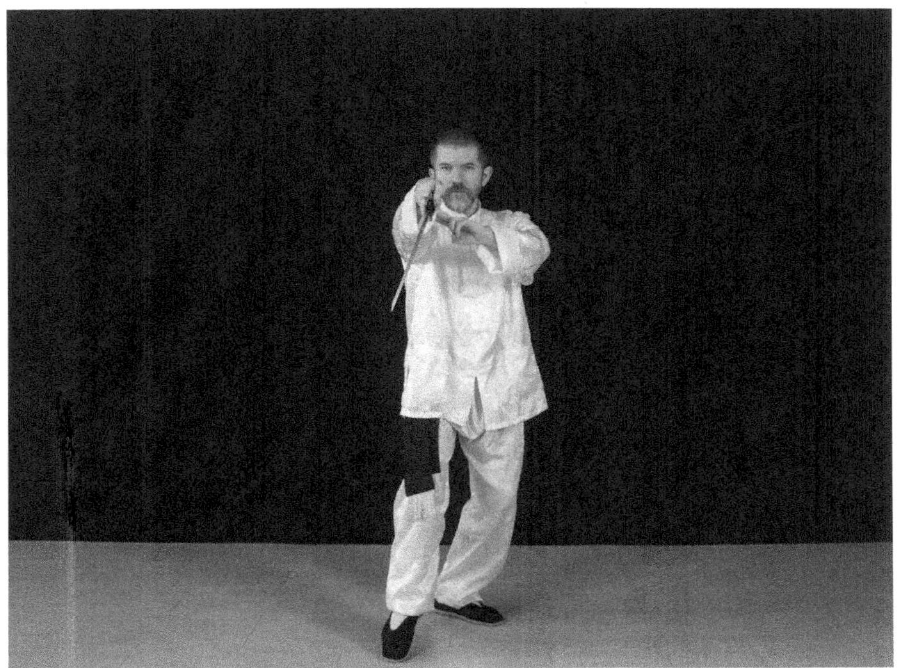

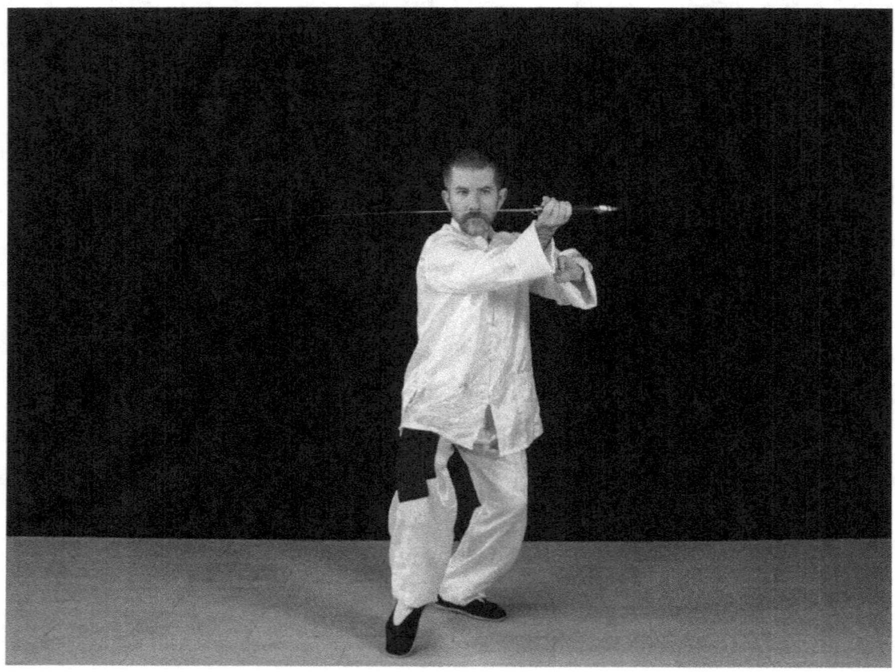

Turn your right wrist ninety degrees to the right to place the sword in the pingmian position. The tip of the blade points west. Then, perform a soft turn of the waist southeast, initiating the movement of the sword. Again, your right wrist should be turned ninety degrees to the left to resume the *zhimian* position.

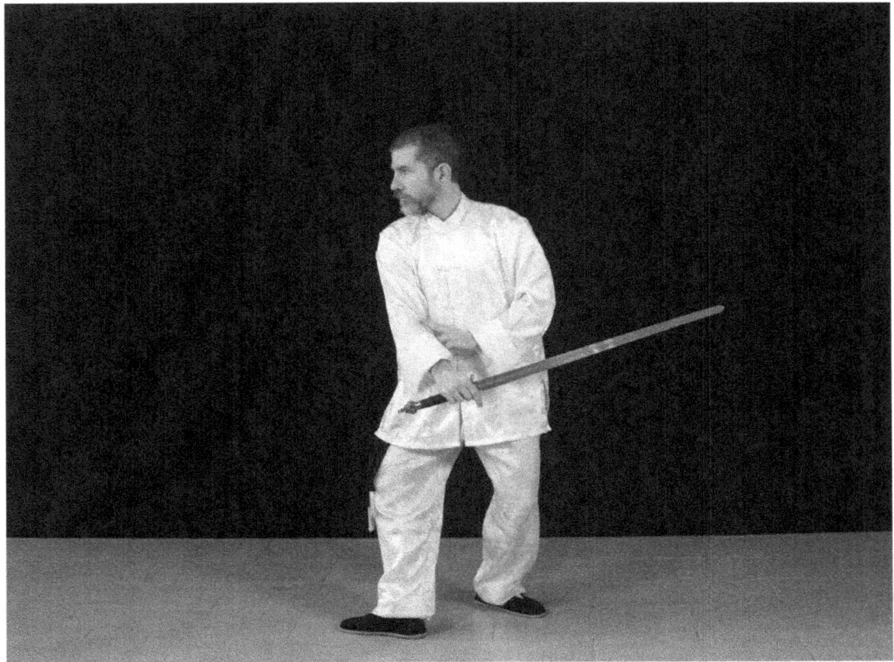

25
Lift up the curtain - 挑帘势

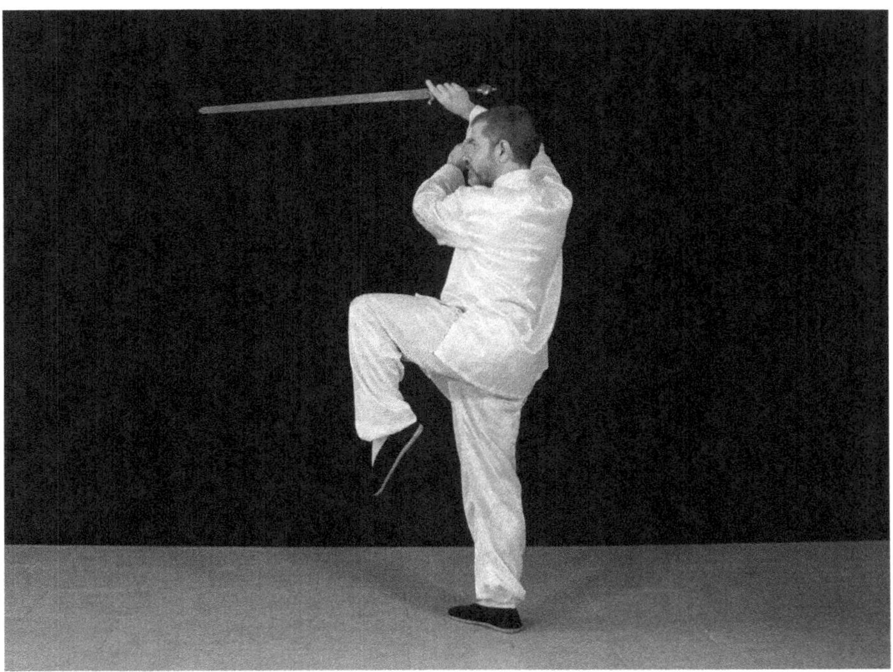

WEST. The sword describes a counter-clockwise ascending arc. At the same time, it is necessary to open your right foot toes until they are facing northwest and turn your waist in the same direction until your torso is facing west. The sword ends up above your head. Keep the balance on your right leg, maintaining your left foot toes towards the ground. The secret sword is kept in the same position throughout the whole technique.

26
Turning the sword to the left - 左輪劍

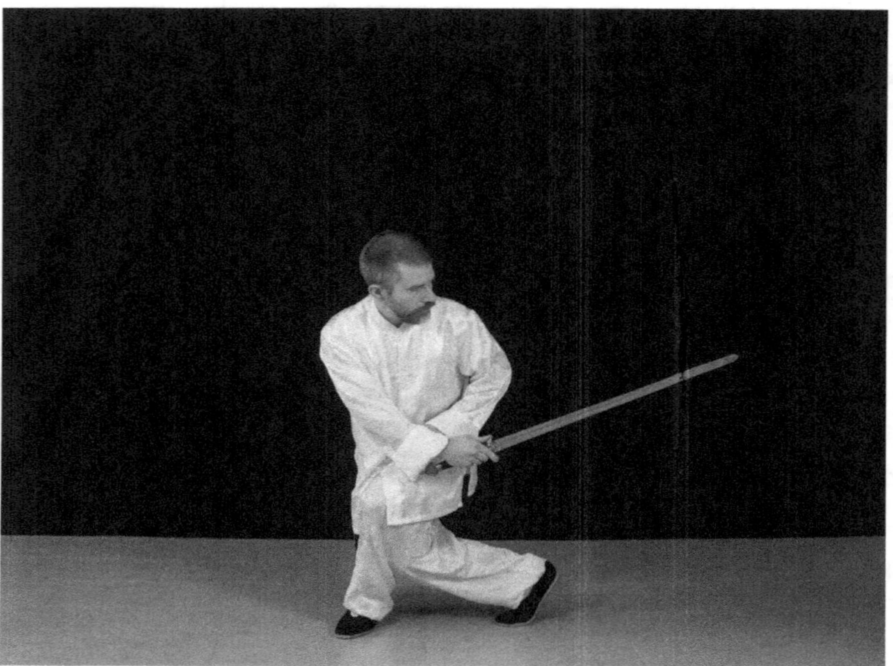

WEST. In this technique, the sword describes a reverse trajectory from that of the previous technique, so as to end its movement executing a thrust to the east from the left flank. The movement of the legs is similar to the nau ma stance, described in the section dedicated to footwork. In order to manage to perform the rotation of the waist correctly, pivot on your left heel, which ends up at the front, until your left foot toes are facing south. Most of the body weight rests on the left leg, and your right knee must be lean against the exterior part of the left gastrocnemius muscle.

27

Turning the sword to the right - 右輪劍

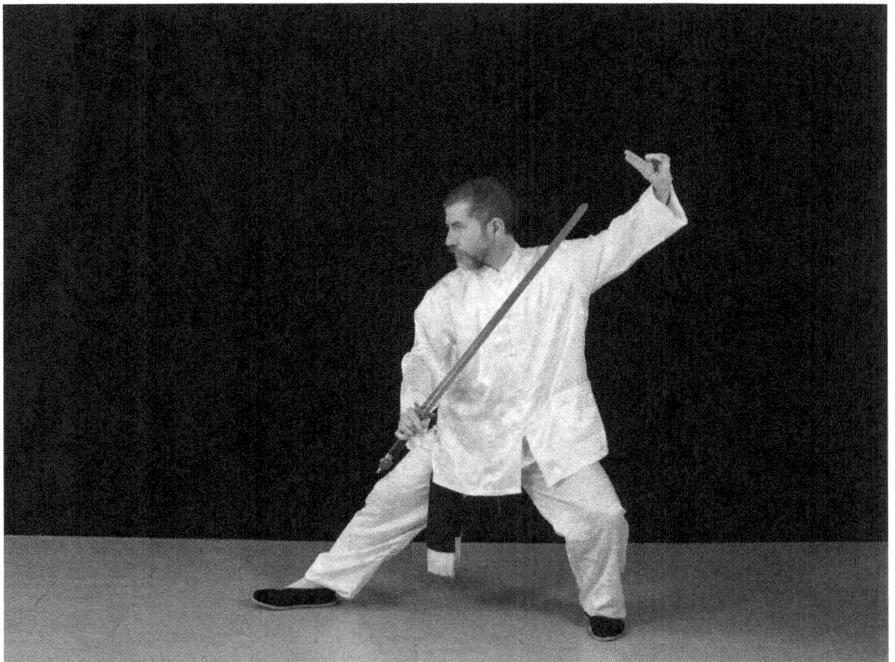

WEST. In the first part of the technique, step into the right bow stance and replicate technique number twenty-three, The comet chases the moon, executing the cut to the west.

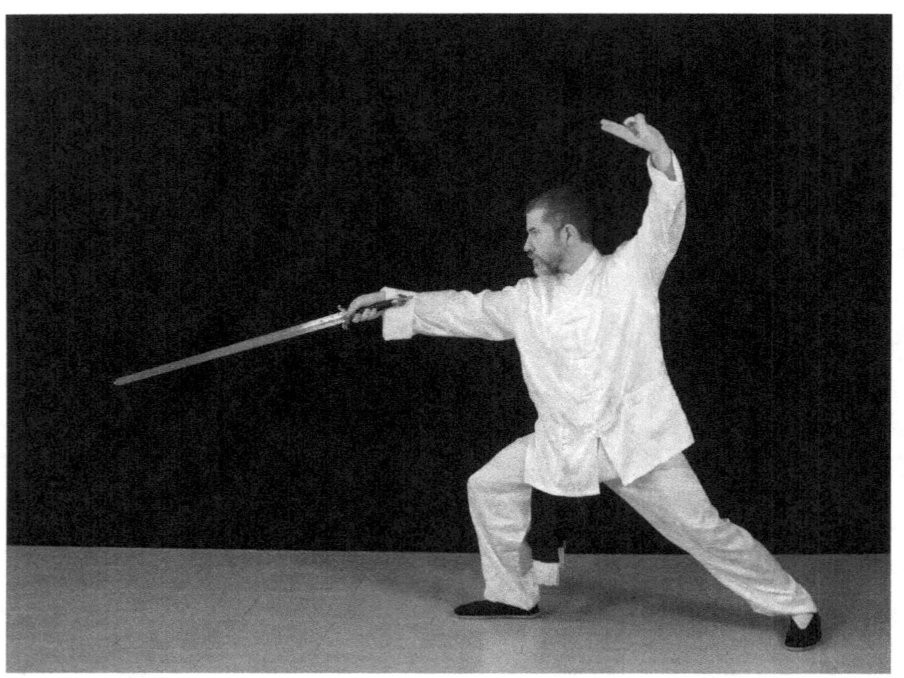

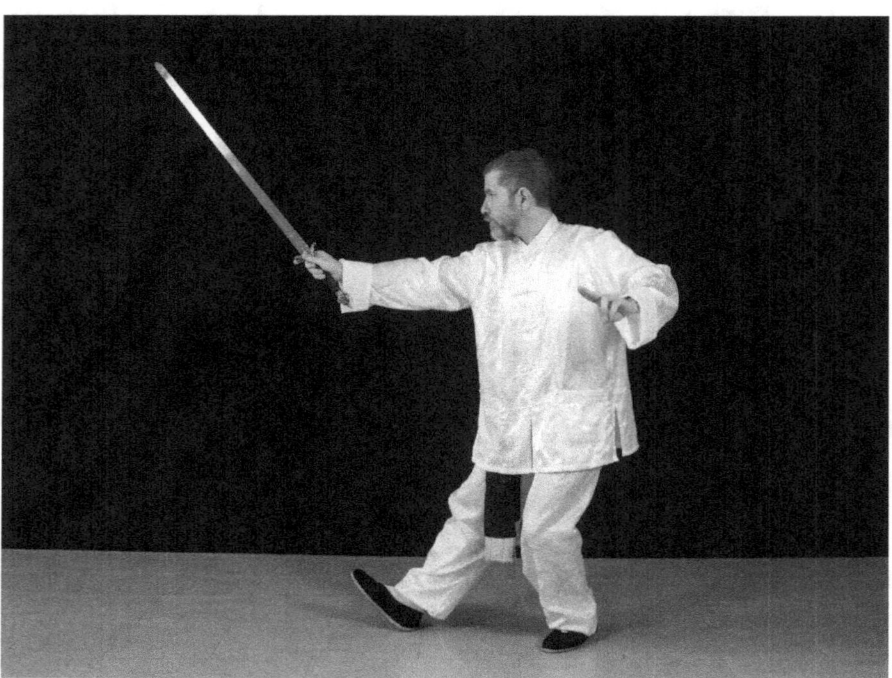

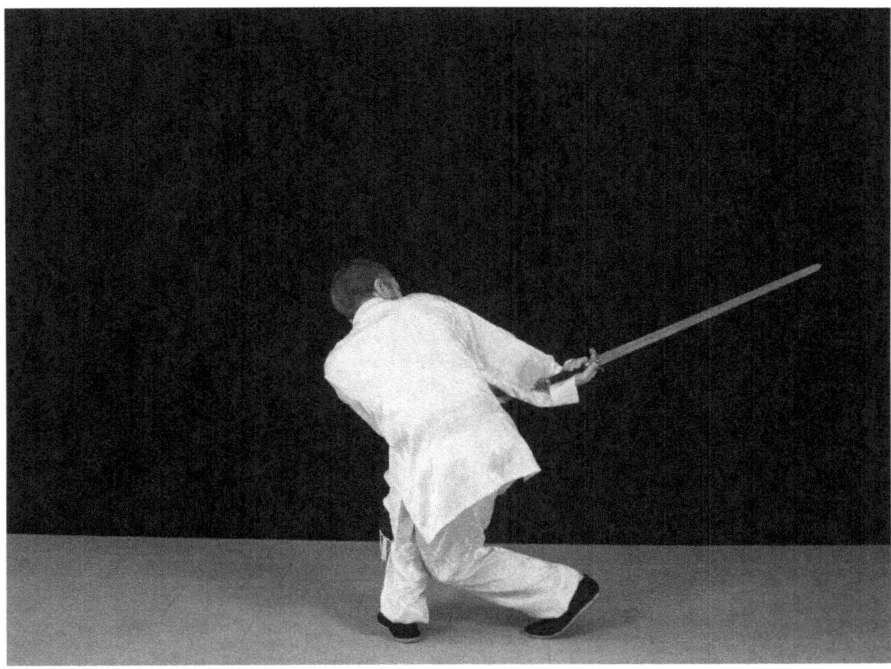

In the second part, step into a stance similar to nau ma, pivoting on your right heel in such a way that your right foot toes are facing north. The sword describes a backward counter-clockwise arc. The point of the blade is directed upwards at a forty-five-degree angle executing a cut to the east from the right flank.

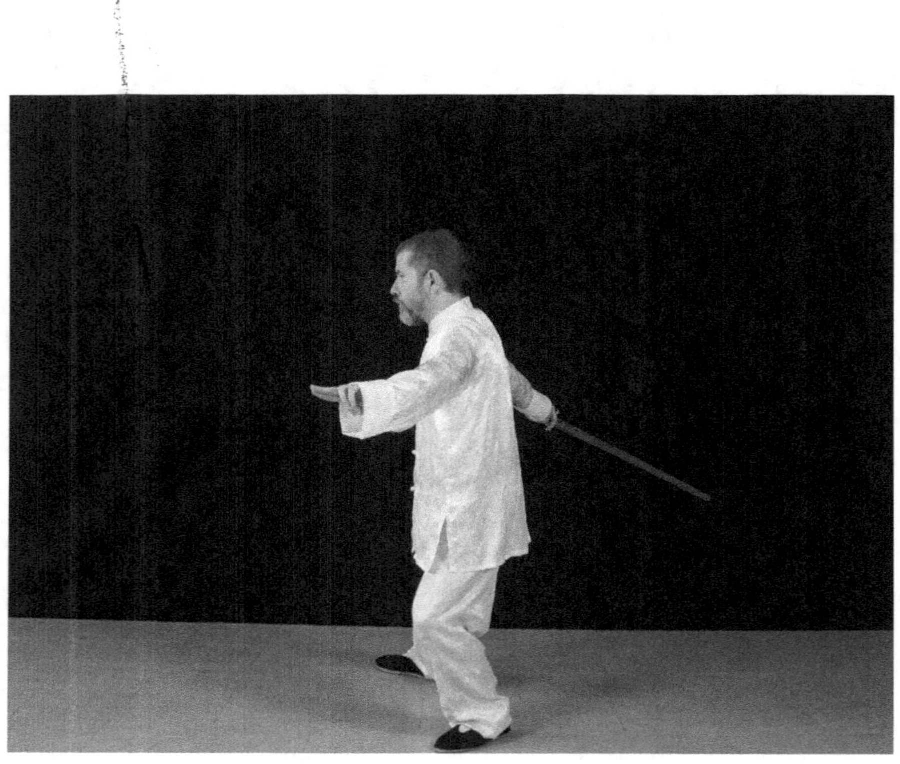

Lastly, advance with your left foot into the middle step of the bow stance, maintaining most of the body weight on your left leg. On this occasion, you should transfer the axis of displacement to the south, opening the width of the step slightly in that direction. In this position, repeat technique number twenty-four, *The celestial horse flies through the waterfall*, executing the cut to the west.

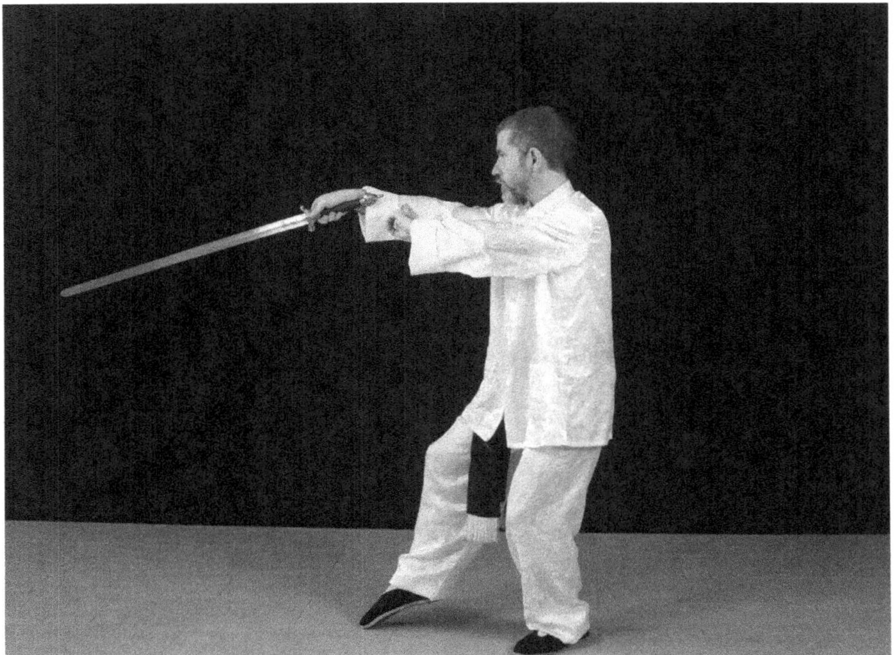

28
The phoenix spreads its wings - 大鵬展翅

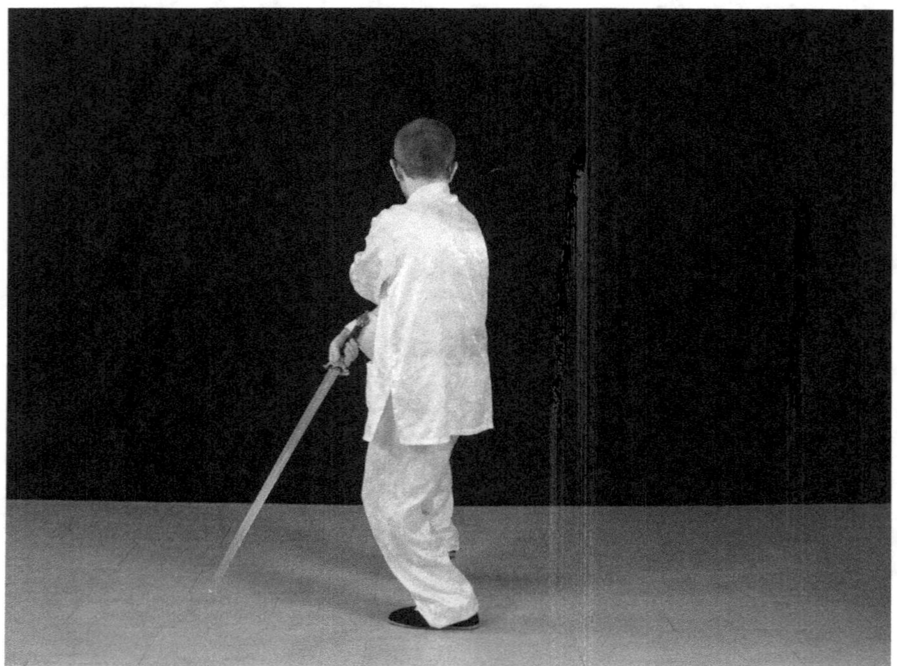

NORTH. Turn your waist until the torso and the toes of your left foot, which pivots on the heel, are facing northwest. The secret sword remains next to your right shoulder, and your right hand is near the left hip. The sword points to the ground at an oblique angle.

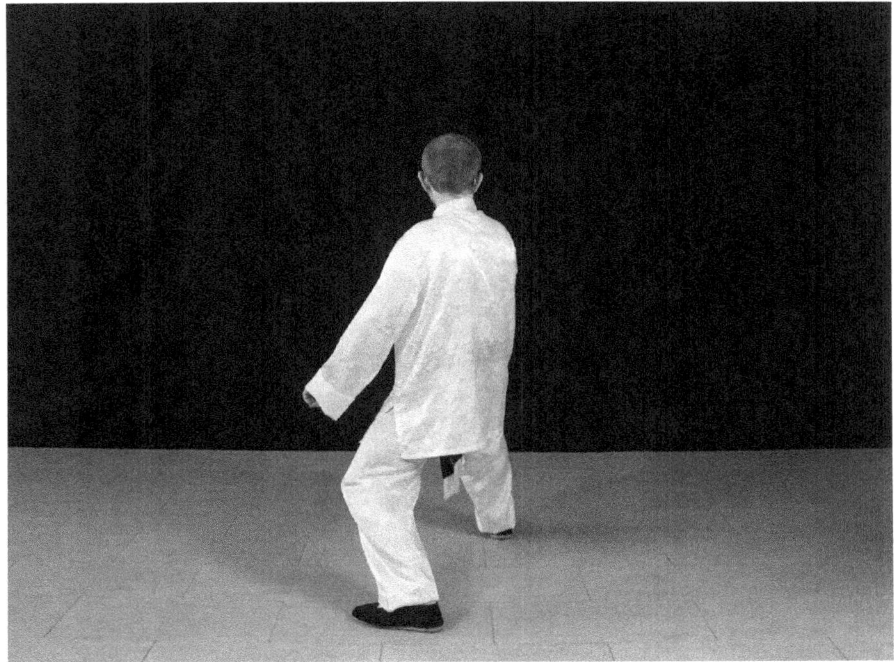

Step into the right bow stance to the north. During the weight shift from the left leg, and the forty-five-degree turn of the waist to the north, the secret sword, with the palm facing down, descends to the left hip and the sword goes up executing a cut in the *pingmian* position up to the height of the right shoulder. The palm of the right hand, which wields the sword, is kept facing up. This technique is equivalent to *Parting wild horse's mane*.

29
The wasp enters the hive - 黃蜂入洞

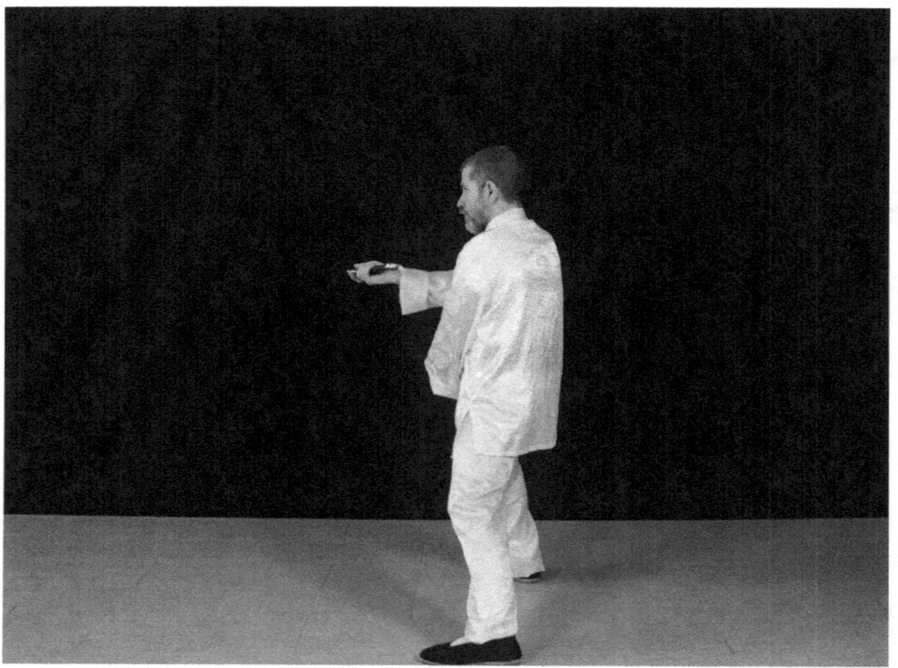

WEST. Place the body weight on your left leg to, immediately after, turn your waist, pivoting on your right heel, until the torso is facing west and your right foot toes are facing northwest. Then, get into the middle step of the bow stance, keeping most of the body weight on your right leg. During this movement, the sword, in the *pingmian* position with the palm of the right hand facing up, performs a circular horizontal counter-clockwise movement that ends with the hilt situated above the right hip. At the same time, the secret sword, oriented likewise, is hidden under the right forearm.

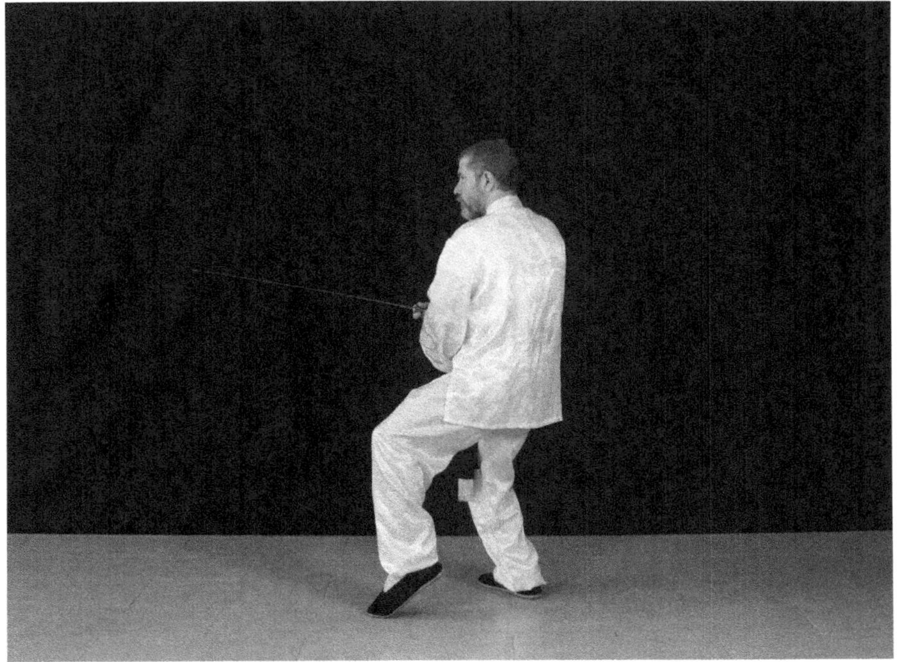

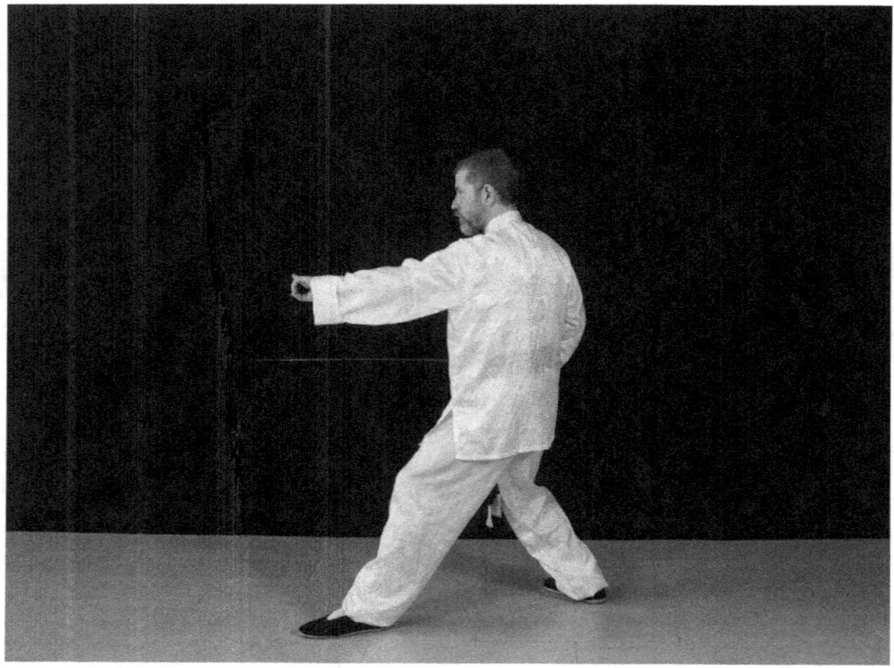

In the second part of the technique, advance with your left foot crossing to step into the right bow stance. The sword executes an ascending recti-linear thrust starting from the hip, in the *pingmian* position. The left hand goes up until it is above the head on the left flank.

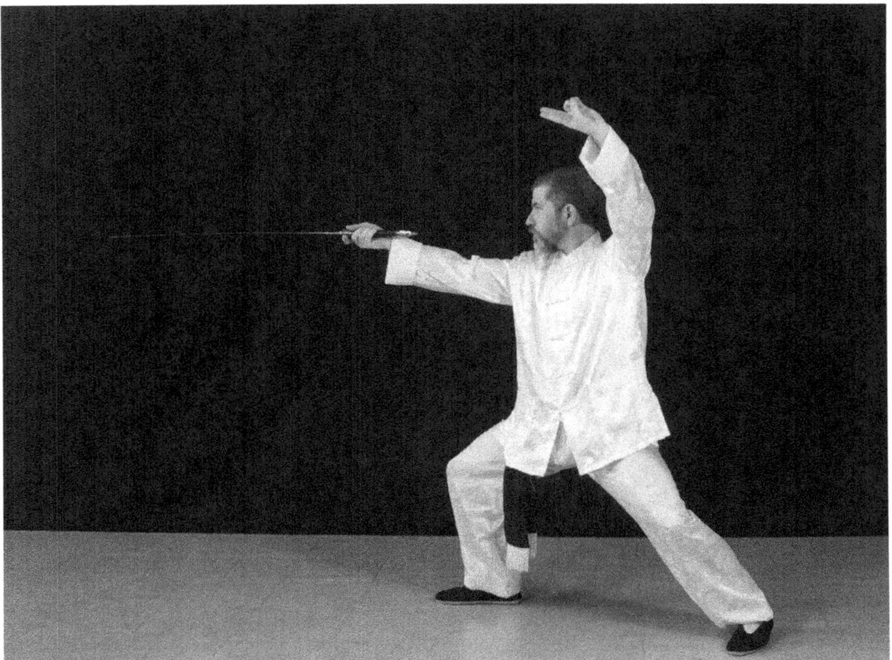

30
Embrace the moon to the bosom - 懷中抱月

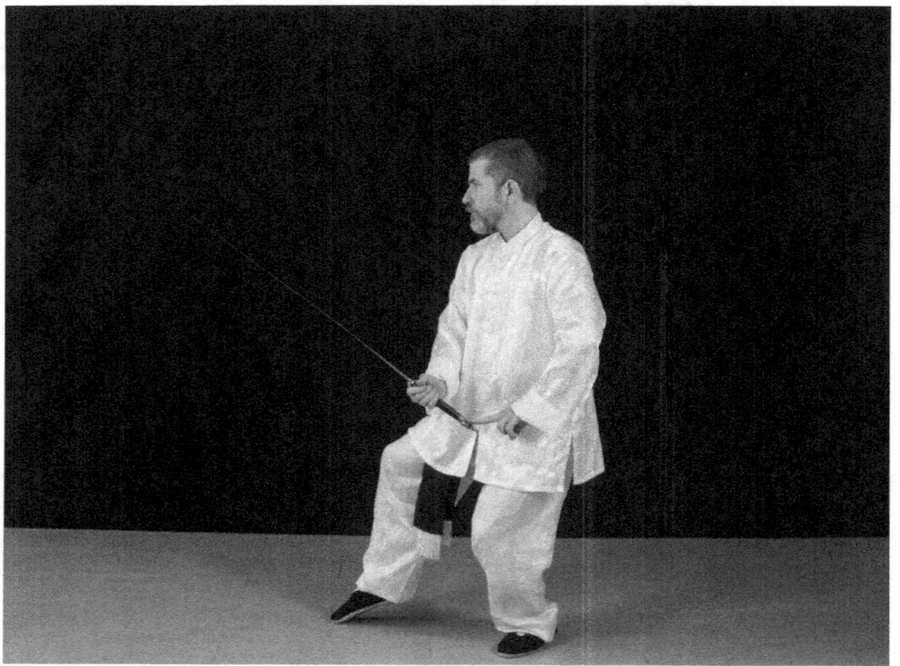

WEST. Resuming the position up to its middle step, replicate technique number seven.

31
The wind sweeps the plum blossoms - 風清掃李子開花

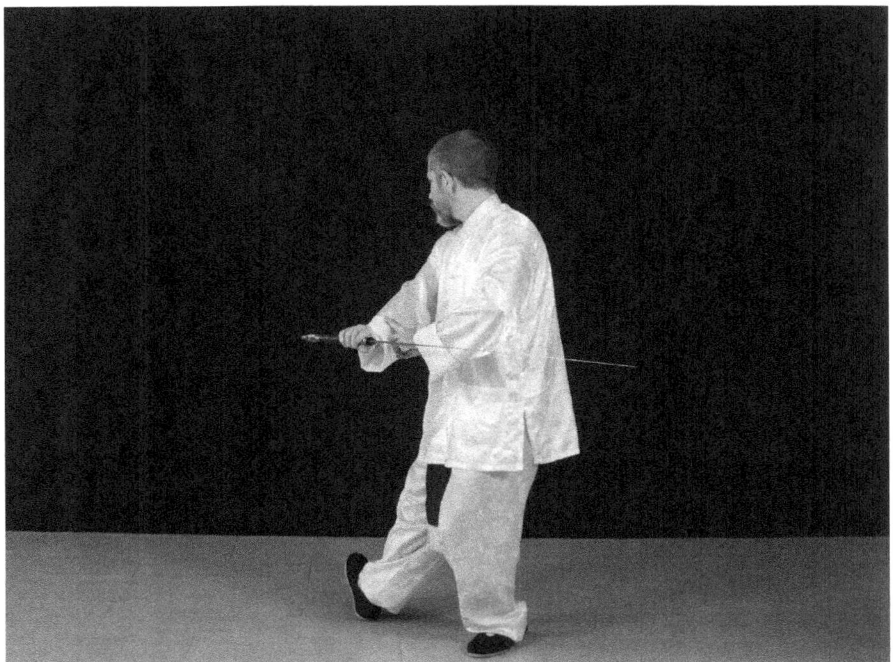

SOUTH. Turn your right wrist so that your palm is face down. The index and middle fingers of the left hand maintain their position on your right forearm. Pivot to the right on your right heel and then place the left foot behind, toes facing southeast. At that point, get into the middle step of the bow stance maintaining the body weight on your left leg. In a similar way to the last part of technique number twelve, *The lion shakes its head*, separate your hands drawing an outward arc starting from the centre of your torso. The tips of the secret sword and the Gim converge at a point in front of your face, forming a triangle.

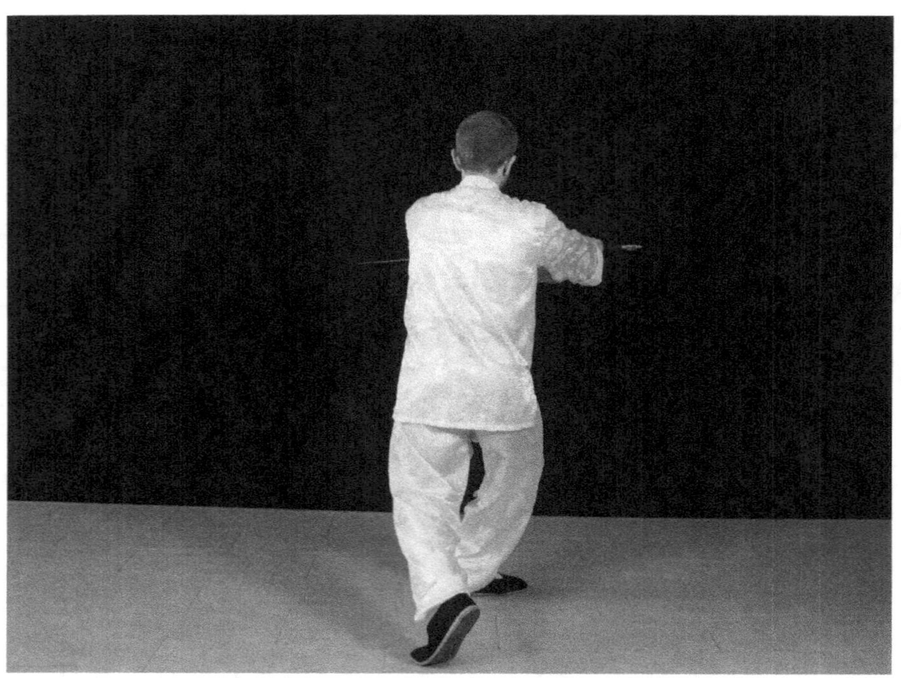

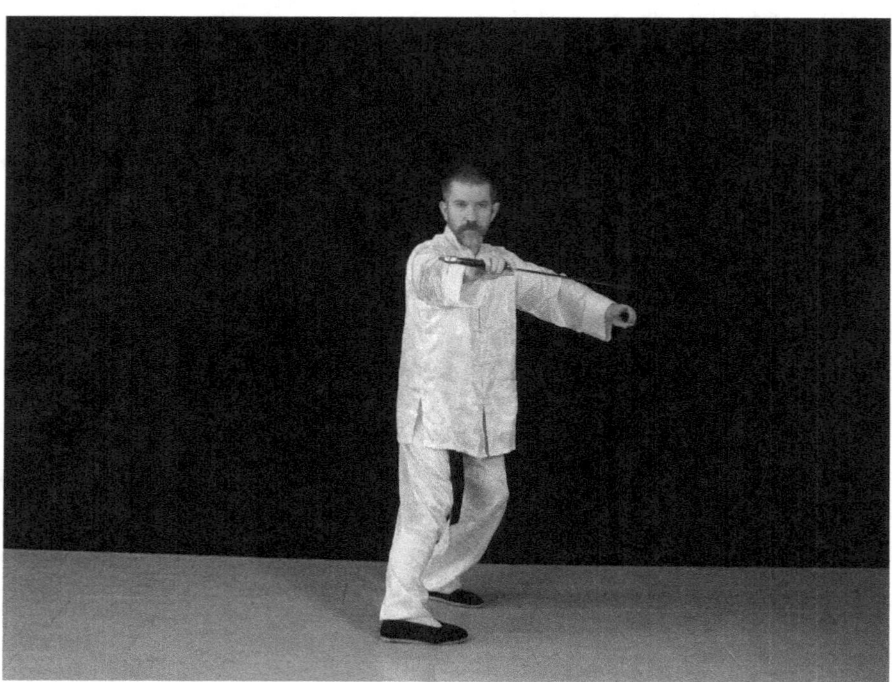

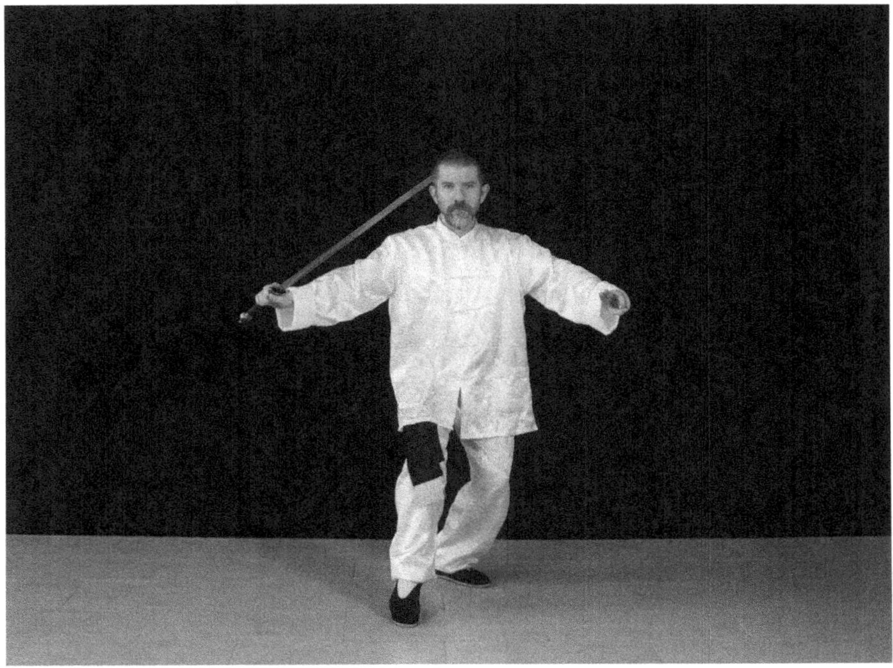

32
The compass needle (points south) - 指南针

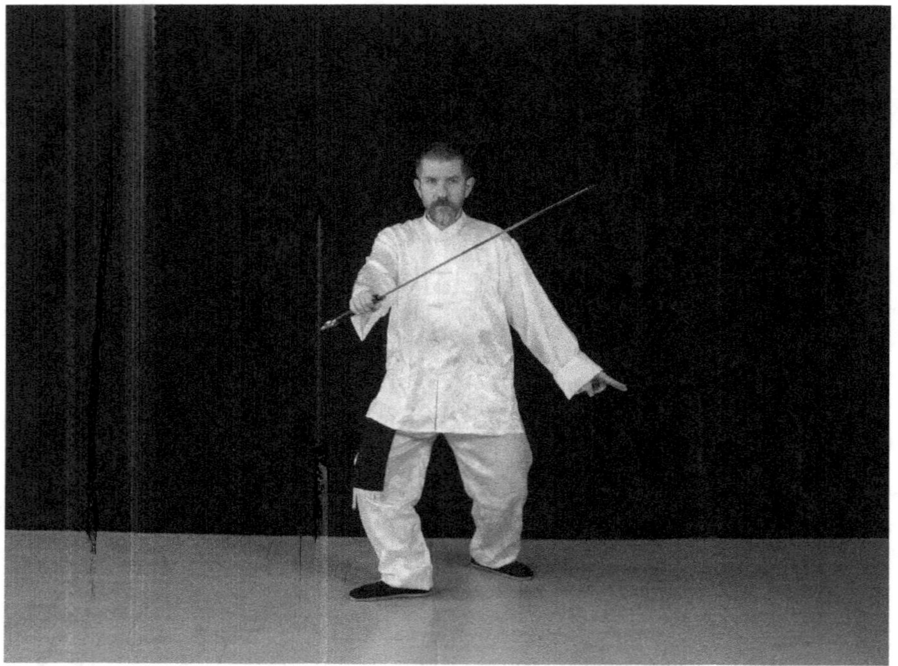

SOUTH. Open your right foot toes crossing the step to allow for the advancement into the left bow stance. Before performing the corresponding weight shift, execute a frontal circular clockwise movement with your left hand, similar to the block with the palm of the hand, or *poon kiu*, while also rotating your waist.

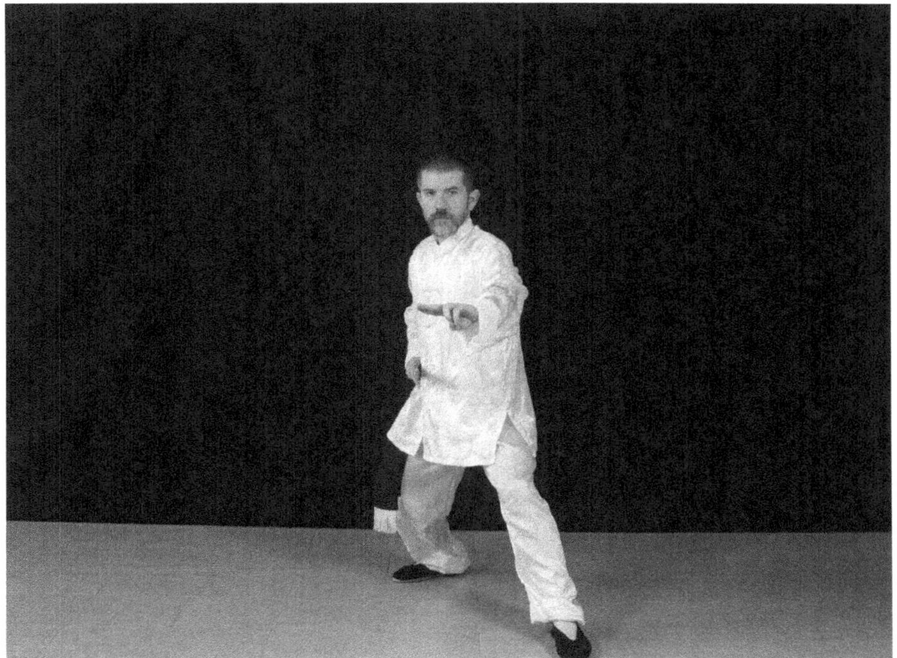

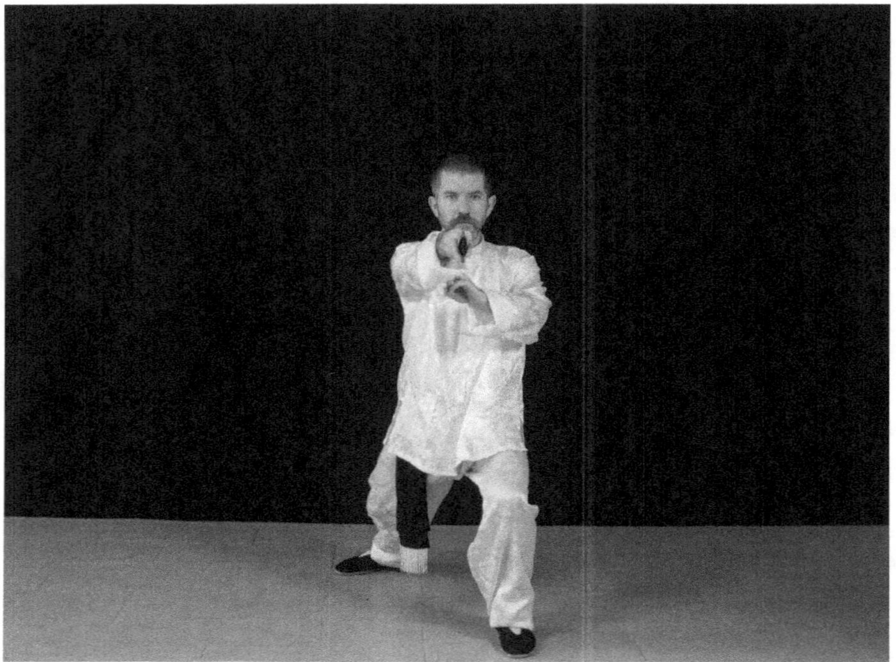

Then, execute a frontal thrust from your right hip, maintaining the sword in the *zhimian* position. The left hand rests close to your right forearm, at a few centimetres from the cubital fossa.

CLOSING

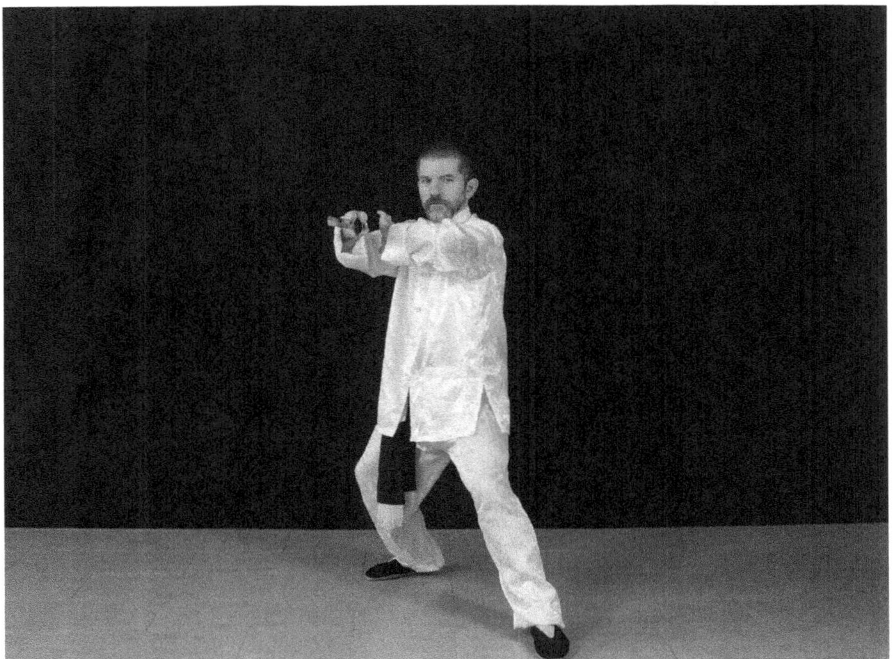

SOUTH. Place most of the body weight on your right leg again. The left hand is placed next to the right ear with the palm facing west. Next, perform a rectilinear movement with your right hand to bring the hilt of the sword closer to the left hand. Hold the sword with your left hand and form the secret sword with the right one. Advance with the right leg, the feet remaining separated at a distance equivalent to the width of your shoulders. The toes are facing south. Bring both hands to the height of the hips, on the sides of your torso.

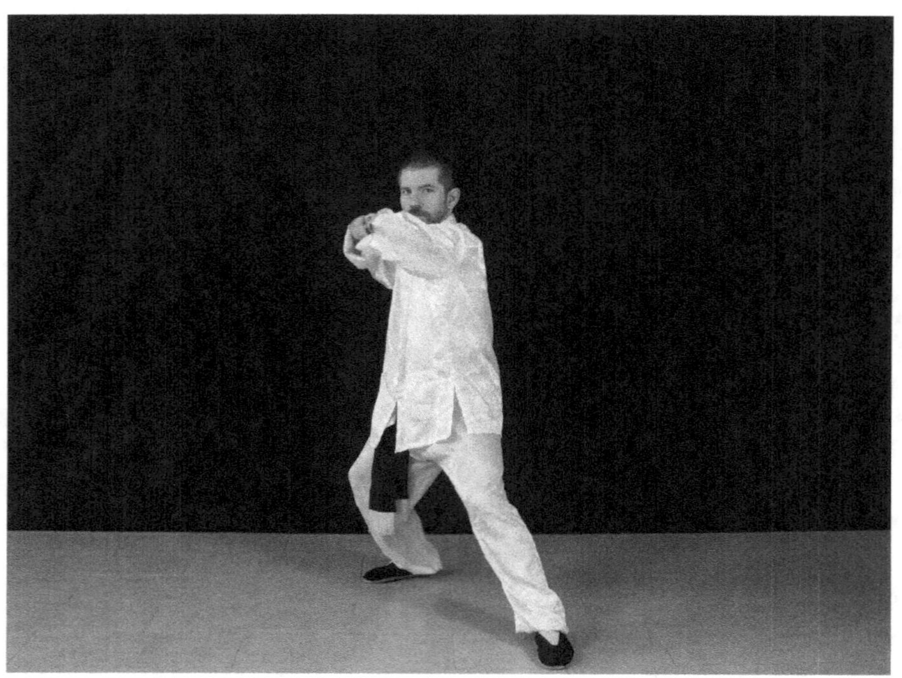

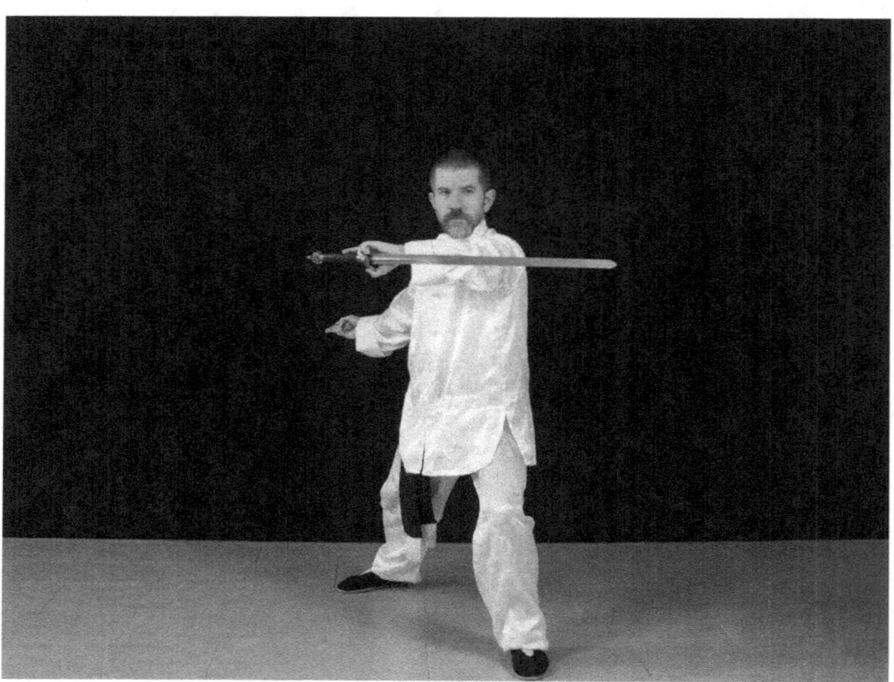

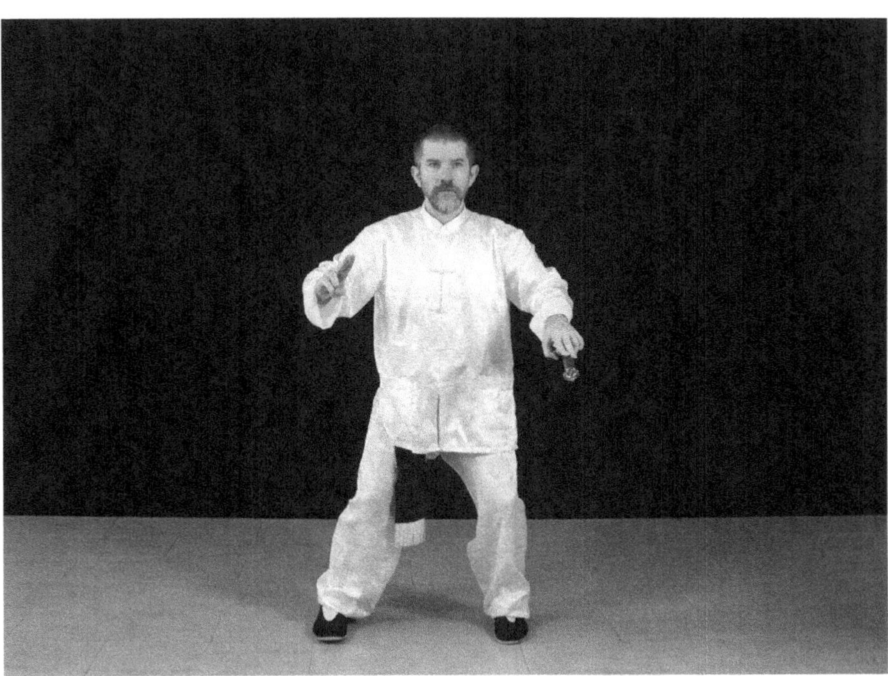

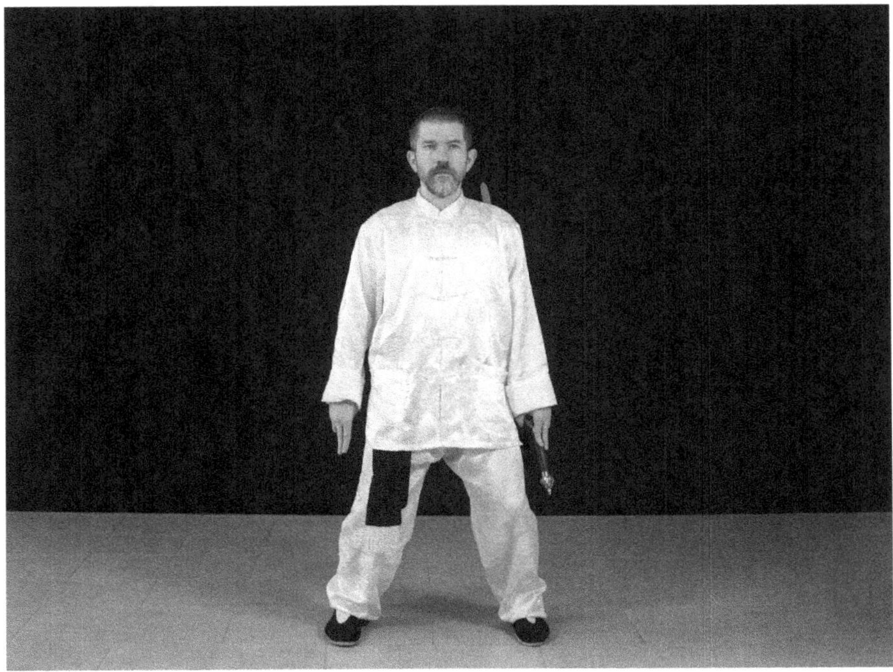

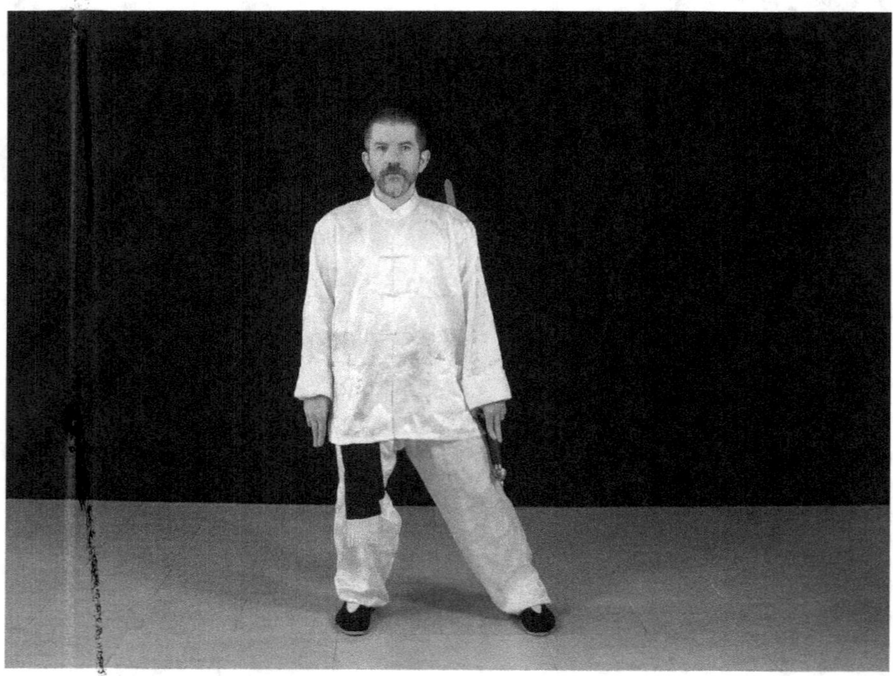

Finally, reverse the sequence of the movements of the opening, placing the body weight on the right leg and bringing the left leg closer. Straighten your knees. Feet close together.

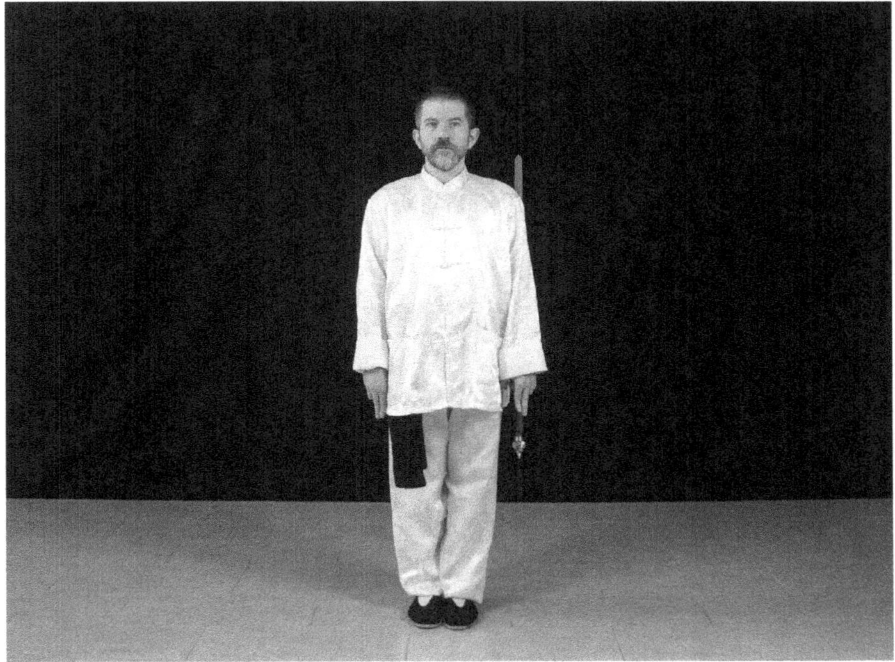

APPENDIX

6
The night demons explore the sea - 夜叉探海

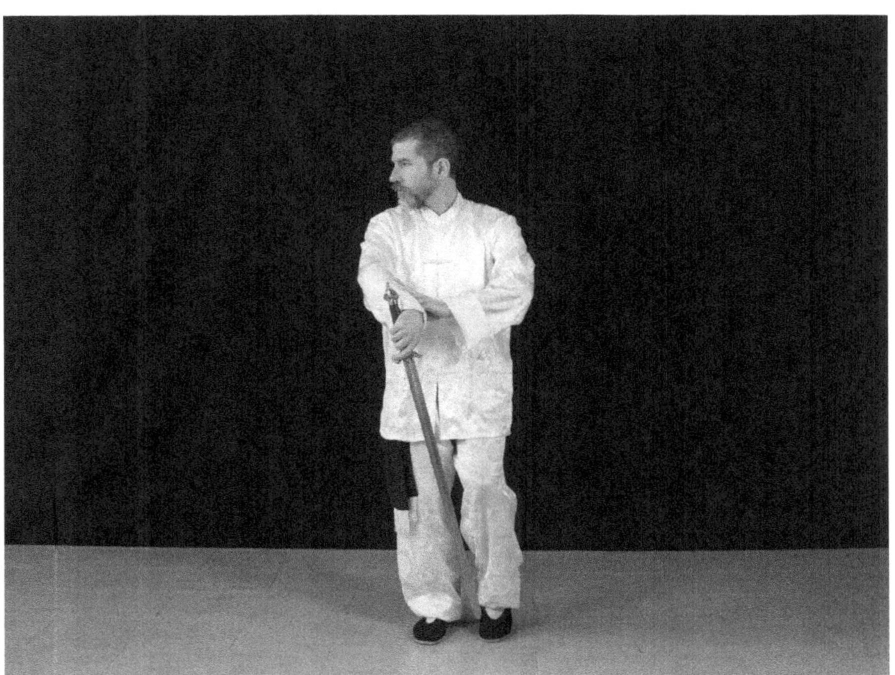

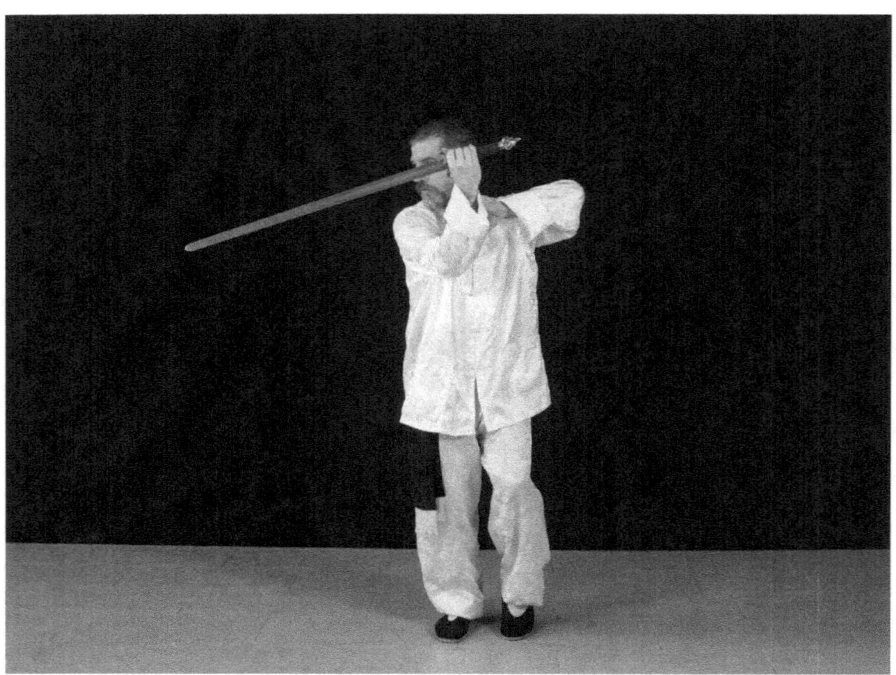

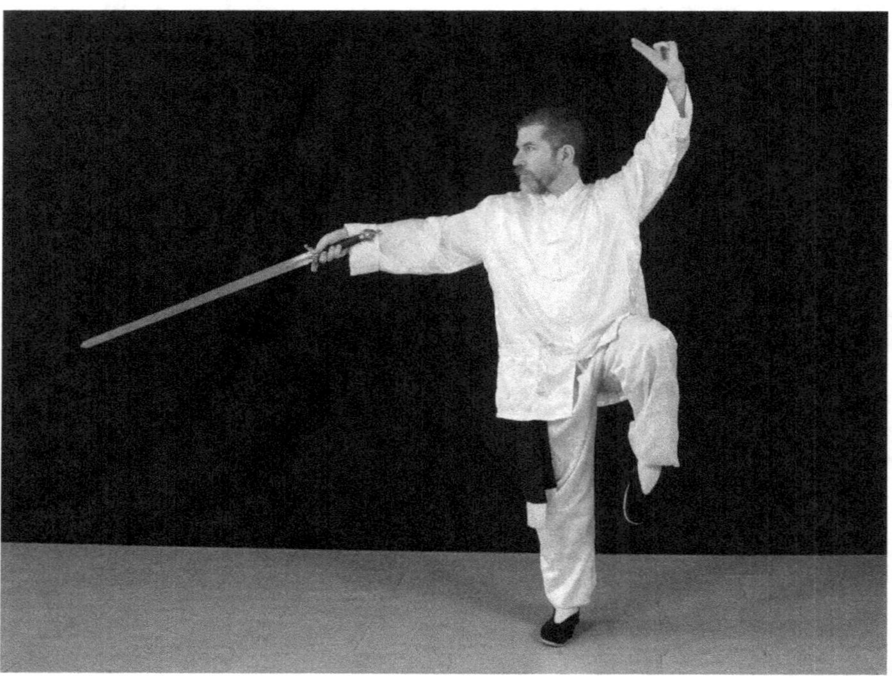

7
Clasping the moon to the bosom - 懷中抱月

8
The sleeping birds return to the forest - 宿鳥投林

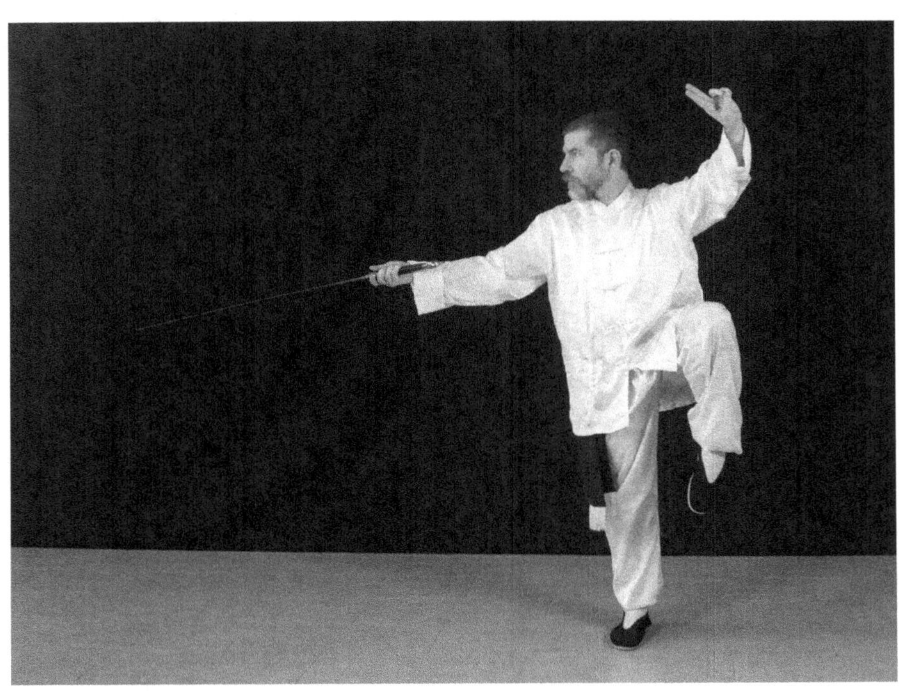

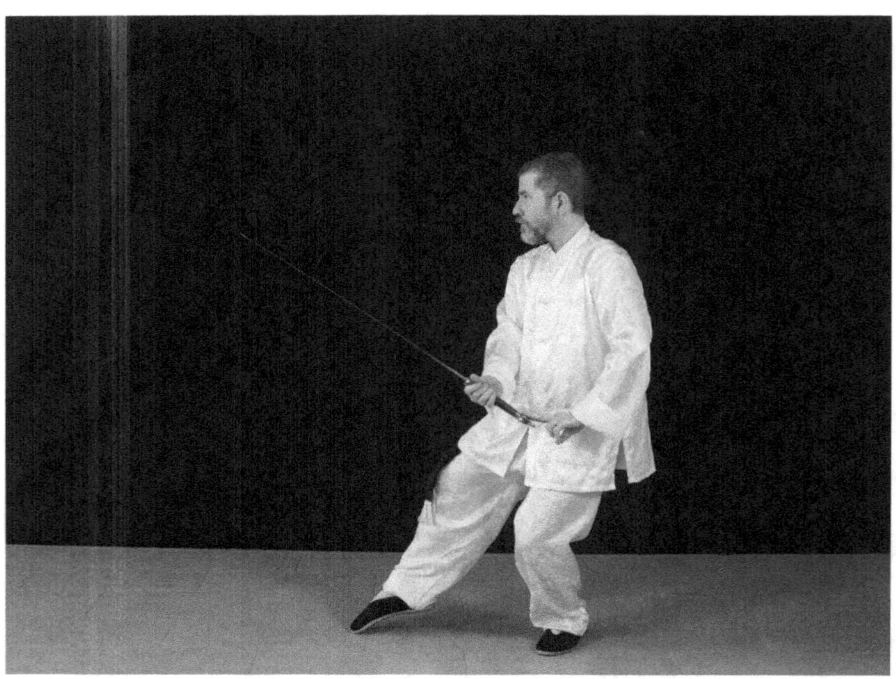

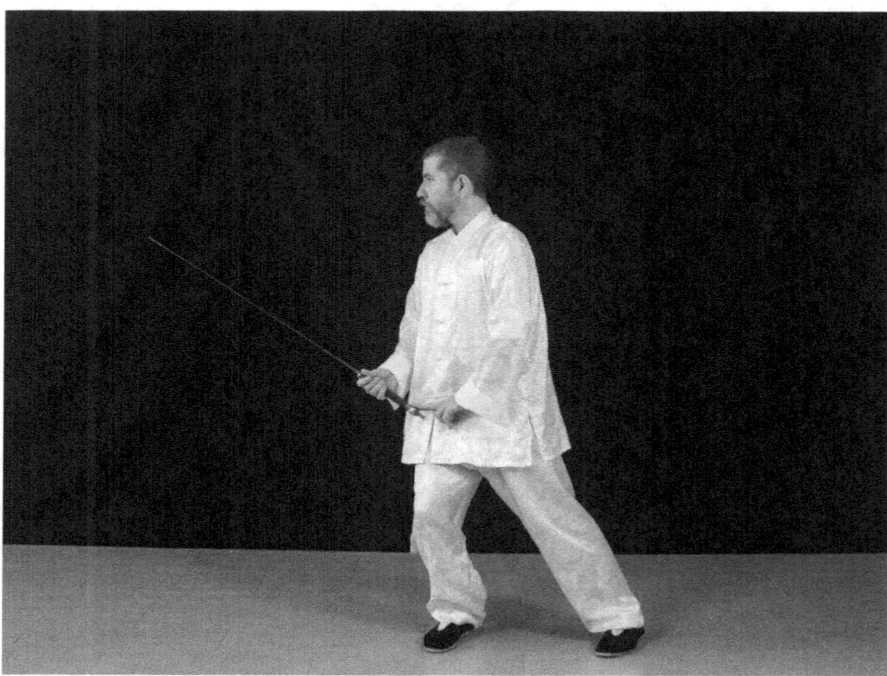

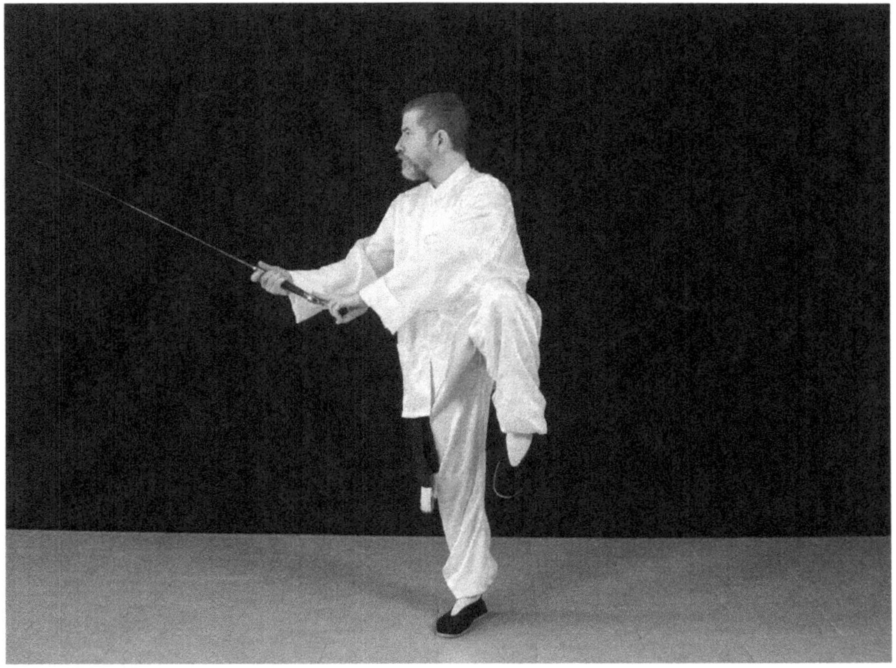

23
The comet chases the moon - 彗星飞行由月亮

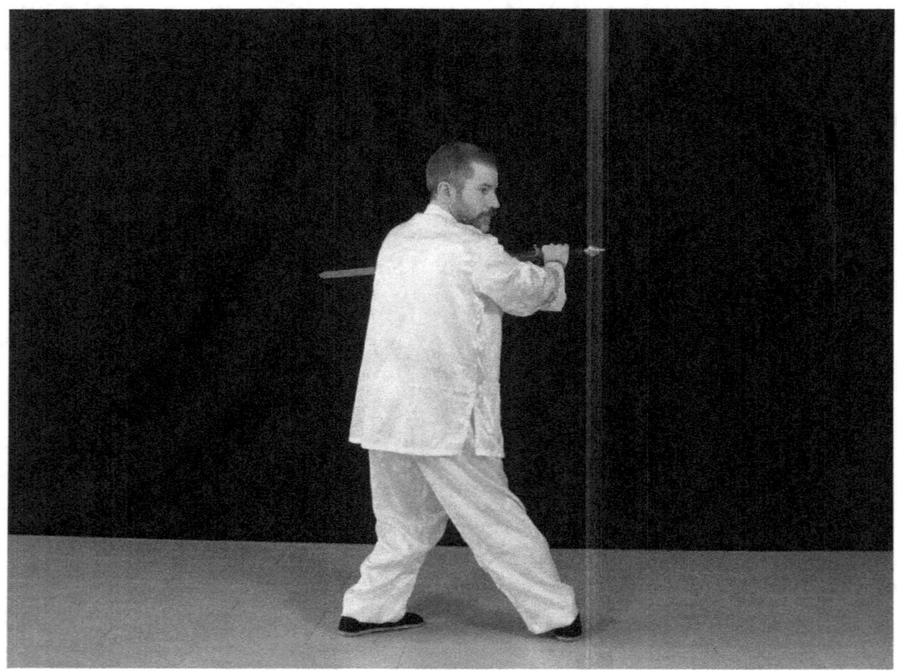

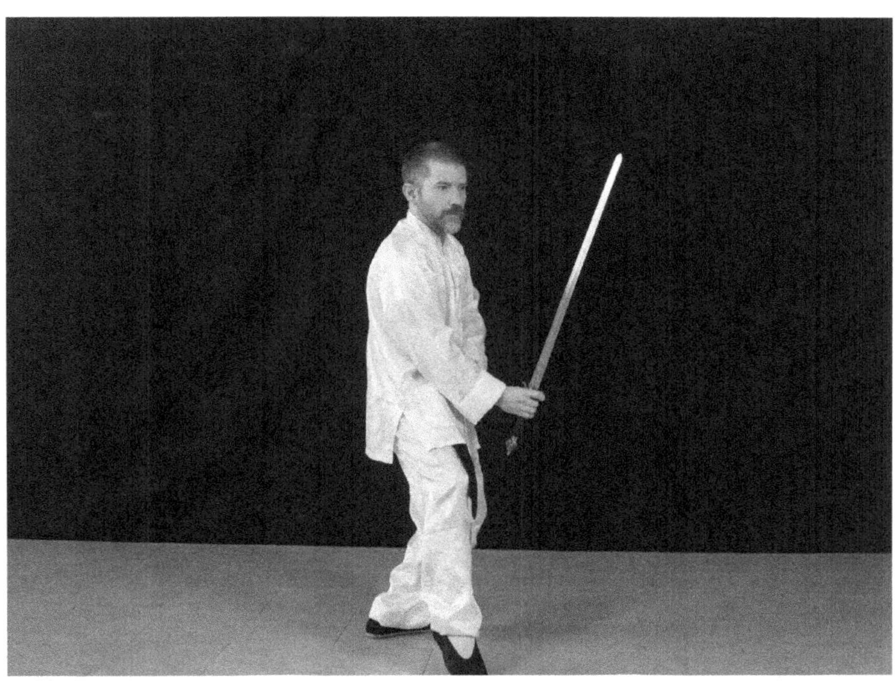

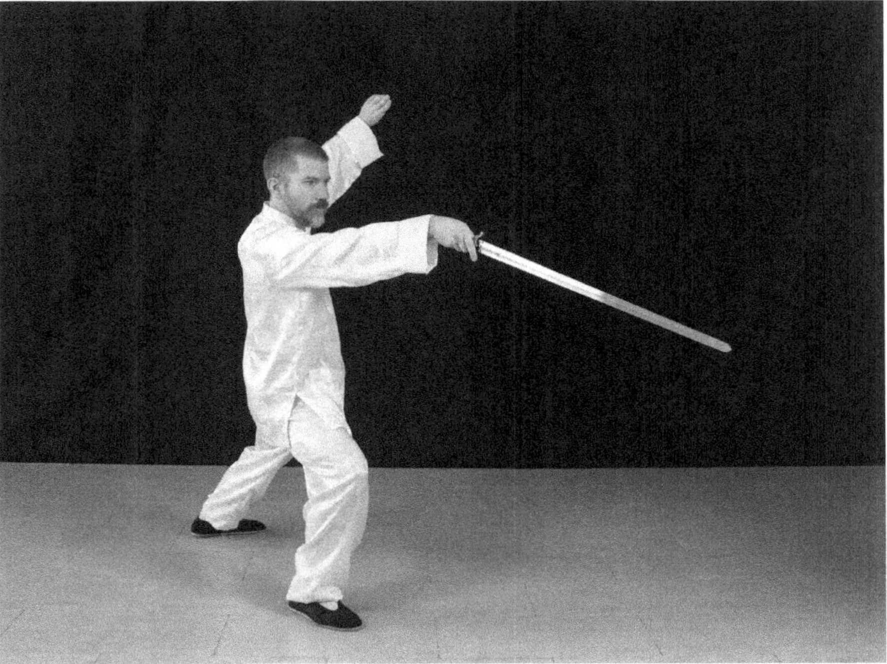

27
Turning the sword to the right - 右輪劍

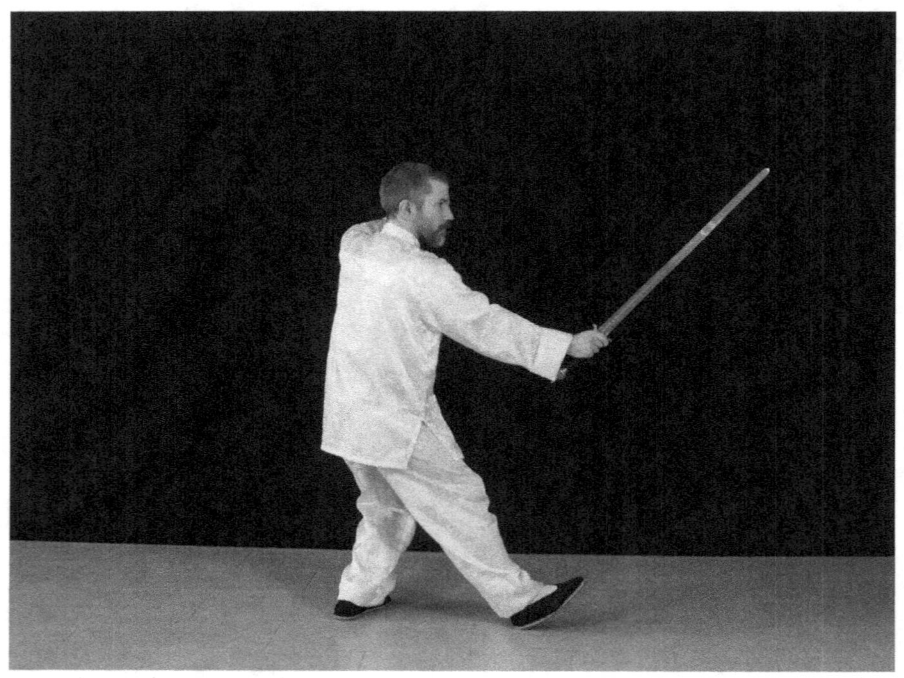

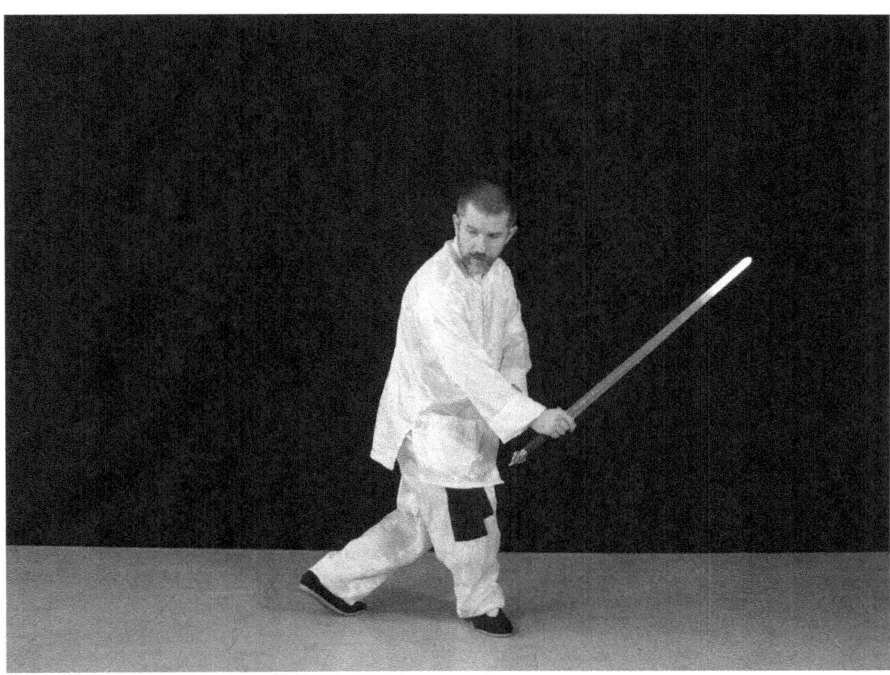

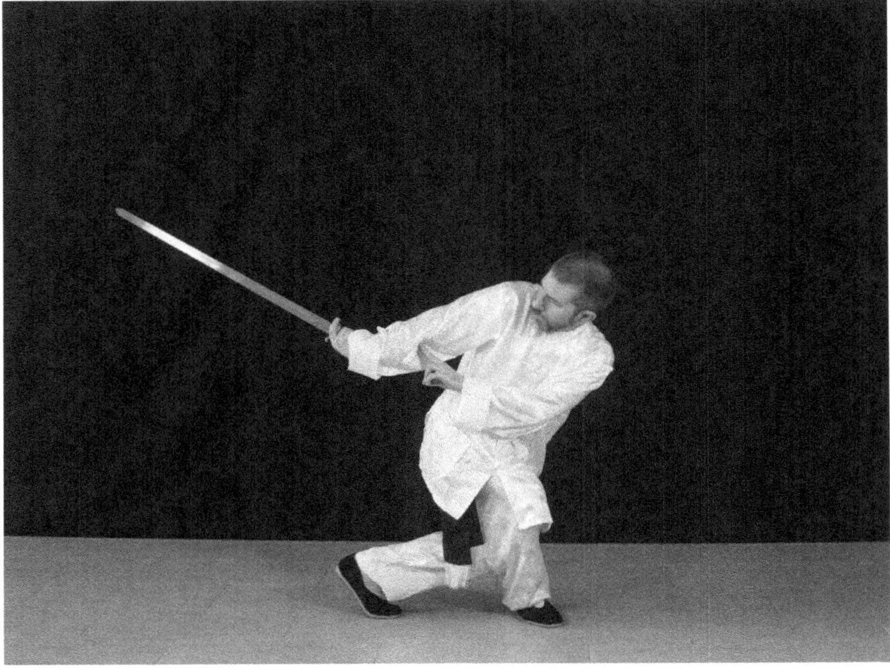

28
The phoenix spreads its wings - 大鵬展翅

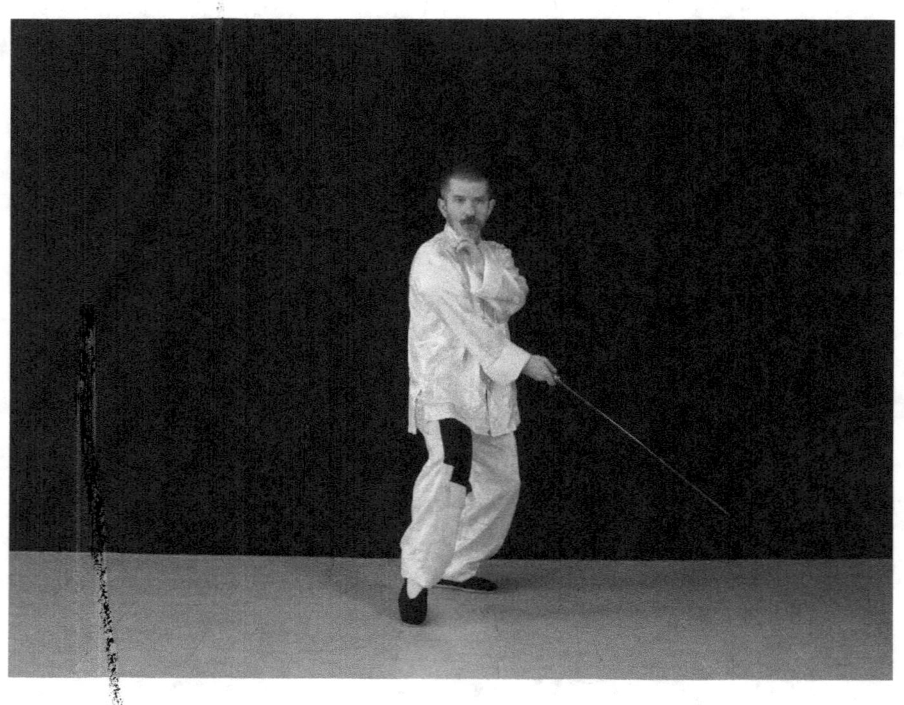

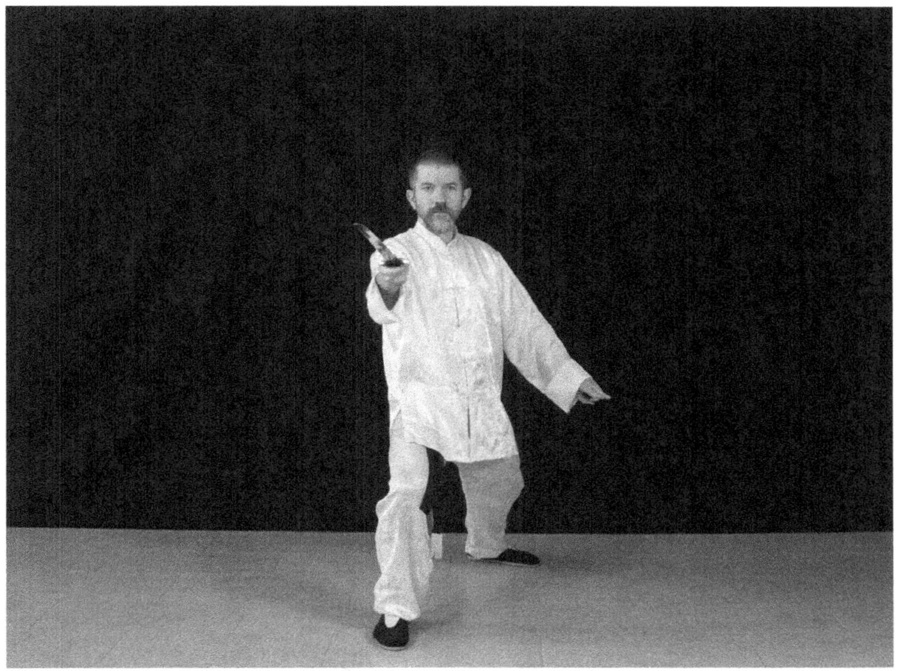

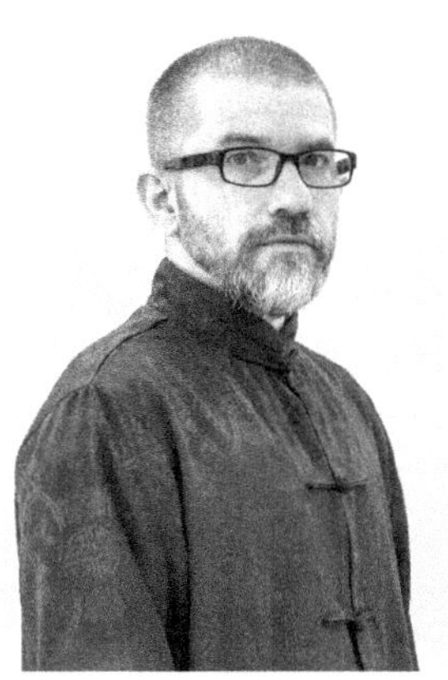

ABOUT THE AUTHOR

Juan Antonio de Blas was trained at the Chinese Martial Arts School of Grandmaster Pedro Rico, one of the most prominent Sifus in Europe; expert in Kung Fu Choy Li Fut and Yang Tai Chi Chuan, and main representative in Europe of the Plum Blossom International Federation, chaired by Grandmaster Doc Fai Wong.

After participating in national and European championships, where he won first awards in different categories of Kung Fu Choy Li Fut and Yang Tai Chi Chuan, Juan Antonio de Blas now focuses his activity on teaching.

Over the years, he has been giving courses and seminars of Tai Chi Chuan, Kung Fu and Chi Kung for both private and public entities, thus contributing in the promotion and conservation of these traditional disciplines.

In close collaboration with the Zaragoza City Council (Spain), Juan Antonio de Blas has taught Tai Chi Chuan and Chi Kung to more than five hundred students each academic term in the last fifteen years.

This informative work is simultaneously complemented by the publication of articles, and the cycle of conferences Martial Arts and Health, which was offered in collaboration with the government of Aragón and the Zaragoza City Council. He is also the author of the books *Tai Chi para personas mayores - un método para mejorar la salud* (in Spanish) and *Kung Fu Choy Li Fut - Wooden dummy 36 step Form*

In order to adapt the traditional performance of Tai Chi, Kung Fu and Chi Kung to the specific needs of different collectives Juan Antonio de Blas sporadically also provides specific courses intended for companies and organizations of diverse natures. In this regard, particular mention may also be made of his work with entities like ASATRA (Aragonese Association for Anxiety Disorder) or CLECE S.A. that provides telecare services for elderly people. Since 2012, he has taught in his own traditional school, Dan Tian, in Zaragoza, Spain.